**Rapid
Obstetrics &
Gynaecology**

RAPID OBSTETRICS & GYNAECOLOGY

Misha Datta
University of Liverpool School of Medicine
Liverpool

Louise Randall
Naomi Holmes
Natasha Karunaharan
All of
Royal Free and University College Medical School
University College London
London

EDITORIAL ADVISORS
Professor Allan MacLean
Consultant
The Royal Free Hospital
London

Mr Paul Hardiman
Consultant
Department of Obstetrics and Gynaecology
The Royal Free Hospital
London

SERIES EDITOR
Amir H. Sam
Royal Free and University College Medical School
University College London
London

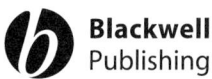

Blackwell
Publishing

© 2003 by Blackwell Publishing Ltd
Blackwell Publishing, Inc., 350 Main Street, Malden, Massachusetts
  02148-5018, USA
Blackwell Publishing Ltd, 9600 Garsington Road, Oxford OX4 2DQ, UK
Blackwell Publishing Asia Pty Ltd, 550 Swanston Street, Carlton, Victoria
  3053, Australia

The right of the Authors to be identified as the Authors of this Work has been asserted in accordance with the Copyright, Designs and Patents Act 1988.

All rights reserved. No part of this publication may be reproduced, stored in a retrieval system, or transmitted, in any form or by any means, electronic, mechanical, photocopying, recording or otherwise, except as permitted by the UK Copyright, Designs and Patents Act 1988, without the prior permission of the publisher.

First published 2003

Library of Congress Cataloging-in-Publication Data

Rapid obstetrics and gynaecology/Misha Datta . . . [et al.].
    p.;   cm.
ISBN 1-4051-1098-8
1 Obstetrics—Handbooks, manuals, etc. 2 Gynecology—Handbooks,
    manuals, etc.
[DNLM: 1 Genital Diseases, Female–Handbooks. 2 Pregnancy
    Complications–Handbooks. 3 Gynecology–Handbooks.
    4 Obstetrics–Handbooks. WQ 39 R218 2003] I. Datta, Misha.
RG110.R37 2003
618—dc21   2002153502

ISBN 1-4051-1098-8

A catalogue record for this title is available from the British Library

Set in 7½ / 9½ pt Frutiger by Kolam Information Services Pvt. Ltd,
  Pondicherry, India
Printed and bound in the United Kingdom by TJ International Ltd,
  Padstow

Commissioning Editor: Vicki Noyes
Editorial Assistant: Nicola Ulyatt
Production Editor: Jonathan Rowley
Production Controller: Kate Charman

For further information on Blackwell Publishing, visit our website:
http://www.blackwellpublishing.com

Contents

Foreword, ix

List of Abbreviations, xi

Rapid Series mnemonic, xiv

Conditions, 1
Adenomyosis, 3
Amenorrhoea, 4
Amniotic fluid embolism, 5
Anaemia in pregnancy, 6
Androgen insensitivity syndrome, 7
Asherman's syndrome, 8
Atrophic vaginitis, 9
Bacterial vaginosis, 10
Bartholinitis, 11
Benign ovarian mass, 12
β-Haemolytic streptococcus—Groups A and B, 14
Candida albicans infection of the genital tract, 15
Carcinoma of the cervix, 16
Carcinoma of endometrium, 17
Carcinoma of ovary, 18
Carcinoma of the vulva, 19
Cardiac disease in pregnancy, 21
Cervical ectopy (erosion) and eversion (ectropion), 22
Cervical intraepithelial neoplasia, 23
Cervicitis, 24
Chlamydia infection of the female genital tract, 25
Chronic hypertension in pregnancy, 26
Chronic pelvic pain syndrome, 27
Diabetes in pregnancy, 28
Dysfunctional uterine bleeding, 29
Dysmenorrhoea, 30
Dyspareunia, 31
Ectopic pregnancy, 32
Endometriosis, 33
Endometritis, 34
Epilepsy in pregnancy, 35
Fetal distress in labour, 36
Fibroids (leiomyomas), 37
Genital warts (condylomata acuminata), 38
Gestational trophoblastic malignancy, 39
Gonorrhoea infection in female genital tract, 40
Hydatidiform mole, 41
Hyperemesis gravidarum, 42
Infertility, 43
Intrauterine death, 45
Intrauterine growth restriction, 46

Kallmann's syndrome, 47
Lichen sclerosus, 48
Malposition, 49
Malpresentation, 50
Mendelson's syndrome, 51
Menopause, 52
Menorrhagia, 53
Miscarriage (spontaneous abortion), 54
Multiple pregnancy, 55
Oligohydramnios, 56
Pelvic inflammatory disease, 57
Placental abruption, 58
Placenta praevia, 59
Polyhydramnios, 60
Polycystic ovarian syndrome, 61
Polyp: cervical and endometrial, 62
Post-coital bleeding, 63
Postmenopausal bleeding, 64
Postnatal blues, 65
Postnatal depression, 66
Post-partum haemorrhage, 67
Pre-eclampsia, 69
Prelabour rupture of membranes, 70
Premenstrual syndrome, 71
Preterm labour, 72
Prolactinoma, 73
Prolonged labour, 74
Prolonged pregnancy, 75
Puerperal psychosis, 76
Puerperal pyrexia, 77
Rhesus isoimmunization (**RhI**) and Rhesus disease (**RhD**), 78
Sexual dysfunction, 79
Sheehan's syndrome, 80
Shoulder dystocia, 81
Thromboembolic disease, 82
Toxic shock syndrome, 83
Trichomonas vaginalis infection of female genital tract, 84
Umbilical cord prolapse, 85
Urge incontinence, 86
Urinary fistula, 87
Urodynamic stress incontinence (previously genuine stress incontinence), 88
Uterine inversion, 90
Uterine rupture, 91
Uterovaginal prolapse, 92
Vaginismus, 93
Vulval intraepithelial neoplasia, 94

Procedures, 95
Amniocentesis, 97
Biophysical profile, 98
Bladder suspension procedures for urodynamic stress incontinence, 99
Caesarean section, 100
Cardiotocograph, 101
Cervical smear, 102
Chorionic villous sampling, 103
Colposcopy, 104
Epidural, 105
Episiotomy, 106
Evacuation of retained products of conception, 107
External cephalic version, 108
Fetal blood sampling in labour, 109
Forceps delivery, 110
Hormone replacement therapy, 111
Hysterectomy, 112
Hysteroscopy, 113
Induction of labour, 114
Laparoscopy, 115
Sterilization (female), 116
Therapeutic abortion, 117
Ultrasonography (in obstetrics and gynaecology), 119
Ventouse delivery, 120

Appendices, 121
Antenatal care, 123
Contraception, 126
Drugs in pregnancy, 129
Infections in pregnancy, 132
Intrapartum care, 137
Postnatal care, 139
Reference ranges, 141

Foreword

As teachers, we expect our students to know everything about our subject. However, it is clearly impossible to retain this huge volume of factual knowledge unless it conforms to some recognisable structure. *Rapid Obstetrics and Gynaecology* provides such a structure. It has been compiled by a group of enthusiastic students who have taken the initiative, identified the areas that require understanding, and liaised with us for our guidance. We have endeavoured to restrict the information to facts with supporting evidence, and avoided areas that are too new or speculative. The result is a fresh approach to learning our subject.

Professor Allan MacLean
Mr Paul Hardiman
January 2003

List of Abbreviations

ABG	Arterial blood gas	CVS	Chorionic villus sampling/ Cardiovascular system
ACE	Angiotensin-converting enzyme	CXR	Chest X-ray
ACRH	Adrenocorticotrophin-releasing hormone	DEXA	Dual energy X-ray absorptiometry scan
ACTH	Adrenocorticotrophic hormone	DHEA	A class of androgen
		DHT	Dihydrotestosterone
ADH	Antidiuretic hormone	DI	Detrusor instability
AF	Atrial fibrillation	D&C	Dilation and curettage
AFP	Alpha feto-protein	DIC	Disseminated intravascular coagulation
APH	Antepartum haemorrhage		
APTT	Activated partial thromboplastin time	DKA	Diabetic ketoacidosis
		DM	Diabetes mellitus
AR	Androgen receptor	DNA	Deoxyribonucleic acid
ARM	Artificial rupture of membranes	DUB	Dysfunctional uterine bleeding
ARDS	Adult respiratory distress syndrome	DVT	Deep vein thrombosis
		ECG	Electrocardiogram
ARF	Acute renal failure	ECT	Electroconvulsive therapy
ASD	Atrioseptal defect	ECV	External cephalic version
AVM	Arteriovenous malformation	EDD	Expected delivery date
AXR	Abdominal X-ray	ELCS	Elective lower segment caesarian section
BA	Bone age		
BCC	Basal cell carcinoma	ELISA	Enzyme-linked *immunoabsorbent* assay
BD	Twice a day		
BMR	Basal metabolic rate	ENT	Ear, nose and throat
BPD	Biparietal diameter	ERPC	Evacuation retained products of conception
BSO	Bilateral salpingo-oopherectomy		
		ESR	Erythrocyte sedimentation rate
BP	Blood pressure		
BV	Bacterial vaginosis	EUA	Examination under anaesthesia
CAH	Congenital adrenal hyperplasia		
		FBC	Full blood count
CBG	Cortisol-binding globulin	FFP	Fresh frozen plasma
CI	Contraindicated	FH(R)	Fetal heart (rate)
CIN	Cervical intraepithelial neoplasia	FISH	Fluorescence *in situ* hybridization
CMV	Cytomegalovirus	FNA	Fine needle aspiration
COC	Combined oral contraceptive	FSH	Follicle-stimulating hormone
CPR	Cardiopulmonary resuscitation	GA	General anaesthetic
		GAGs	Glycosaminoglycans
CRF	Corticotrophin-releasing factor	GDM	Gestational diabetes mellitus
		GFR	Glomerular filtration rate
CRH	Cortisol-releasing hormone	GH	Growth hormone
CRL	Crown–rump length	GHRH	Growth-hormone-releasing hormone
CRP	C-reactive protein		
CS	Caesarian section	GI	Gastrointestinal
CSF	Cerebrospinal fluid	GIFT	Gamete intrafallopian transfer
CT	Computerized tomography		
CTG	Cardiotocograph	GnRH	Gonadotrophin-releasing hormone
CVA	Cerebovascular accident		
CVP	Central venous pressure	GSI	Genuine stress incontinence

GTT	Glucose tolerance test	LH	Luteinizing hormone/ Laparoscopic hysterectomy
Hb	Haemoglobin		
hCG	Human chorionic gonadotrophin	LLETZ	Large loop excision of transformation zone
HDL	High-density lipoprotein	LMP	Last menstrual period
HELLP	Haemolysis, elevated liver enzymes, low platelets	LMW	Low molecular weight
		LN	Lymph node
		LSCS	Lower segment caesarian section
HH	Hypogonadotrophic hypogonadism	MAO	Monoamine oxidase
HPO	Hypothalamus pituitary ovary (as in axis)	MCV	Mean cell volume
		MEN	Multiple endocrine neoplasia
HPV	Human papilloma virus	MI	Myocardial infarct
HR	Heart rate	MIF	Müllerian-inhibiting factor
HRT	Hormone replacement therapy	MM	Malignant melanoma
		MRI	Magnetic resonance imaging
HVS	High vaginal swab	MSU	Midstream urine
ICP	Intracranial pressure	NFPA	Non-functioning pituitary adenoma
ICSI	Intracytoplasmic sperm injection		
		NSAIDs	Non-steroidal anti-inflammatory drugs
IDDM	Insulin-dependant diabetes mellitus		
		NTD	Neural tube defect
Ig	Immunoglobulin	OCP	Oral contraceptive pill
IGT	Impared glucose tolerance	OGTT	Oral glucose tolerance test
IHD	Ischaemic heart disease	PCB	Post-coital bleeding
IM	Intramuscular	PCO	Polycystic ovaries
IMB	Intermenstrual bleed	PCOS	Polycystic ovarian syndrome
IOL	Induction of labour	PCR	Polymerase chain reaction
IPPV	Intermittent positive pressure ventilation	PCV	Packed cell volume
		PDA	Patent ductus arteriosis
ITT	Insulin tolerance test	PE	Pulmonary embolism
ITU	Intensive therapy unit	PG	Prostaglandin
IUCD	Intrauterine contraceptive device	PID	Pelvic inflammatory disease
		PIH	Pregnancy-induced hypertension
IUD	Intrauterine death		
IUGR	Intrauterine growth restriction	PMB	Postmenopausal bleed
		PMS	Premenstrual syndrome
IUS	Intrauterine system	PO	Per os (orally)
IV	Intravenous	POP	Progesterone-only pill
IVF	*In vitro* fertilization	PPH	Post-partum haemorrhage
IVP	Intravenous pyelogram	PR	Per rectum
IVU	Intravenous urogram	PRL	Prolactin
Ix	Investigations	PROM	Prelabour rupture of membranes
JVP	Jugular venous pressure		
KAL	A specific gene when mutated causes GnRH deficiency	PTU	Propylthiouracil
		PV	Per vaginum
		RFT	Renal function tests
LCR	Ligase chain reaction	Rh	Rhesus
LDL	Low-density lipoprotein	RhD	Rhesus disease
LFT	Liver function test	RhI	Rhesus isoimmunization
LGA	Large for gestational age	ROM	Rupture of membranes

RUQ	Right upper quadrant	TSH	Thyroid-stimulating hormone
SC	Subcutaneous	TSS	Trans-sphenoidal selective adenomectomy
SCC	Squamous cell carcinoma		
SE	Side effects	TV	Transvaginal
SHBG	Sex-hormone-binding globulin	TVT	Tension-free vaginal tape
		UA	Urinanalysis
SIADH	Syndrome of inappropriate ADH	U&E	Urea and electrolytes
		US	Upper segment (reference to bone length)
SLE	Systemic lupus erythematosus		
		USI	Urodynamic stress incontinence
SOB	Short of breath		
SRM	Spontaneous rupture of membranes	USS	Ultrasound scan
		UTI	Urinary tract infection
SSRI	Selective serotonin reuptake inhibitor	VC	Verrucous carcinoma
		VDRL	Venereal disease research laboratory
STI	Sexually transmitted infection		
		VE	Vaginal examination
SXR	Skull X-ray	VH	Vaginal hysterectomy
TAH	Total abdominal hysterectomy	VIN	Vaginal intraepithelial neoplasia
TB	Tuberculosis	VIP	Vasoactive intestinal polypeptide
TBG	Thyroid-binding globulin		
TBPA	Thyroid-binding pre-albumin	VLDL	Very low-density lipoprotein
TED	Thromboembolic disease	VQ	Ventilation : perfusion ratio
TENS	Transcutaneous electrical nerve stimulation	VSD	Ventriculo-septal defect
		WCC	White cell count
TES	Transethmoidal selective adenomaectomy	WHO	World Health Organization
		WLE	Wide local excision
TFT	Thyroid function test		
TH	Thyroid hormone	**SYMBOLS**	
TIA	Transient ischaemic attack	>	Less than
TIBC	Total iron-binding capacity	<	Greater than
TOP	Termination of pregnancy	/	Or
TPHA	*Trepenoma pallidum* haemagglutination	↑	Increased
		↓	Decreased
TPN	Total parenteral nutrition	→	Results in
TPO	Thyroid peroxidase	?	Possible/possibly
TRH	Thyroid-releasing hormone		

Rapid Series mnemonic

CONDITIONS
- **D:** Definition — *Doctors*
- **A:** Aetiology — *Are*
- **A/R:** Associations/Risk factors — *Always*
- **E:** Epidemiology — *Emphasizing*
- **H:** History — *History taking &*
- **E:** Examination — *Examining*
- **P:** Pathology — *Patients*
- **I:** Investigations — *In*
- **M:** Management — *Managing*
- **C:** Complications — *Clinical*
- **P:** Prognosis — *Problems*

PROCEDURES
- **D:** Definition
- **I:** Indications
- **M:** Method
- **A:** Advantages
- **D:** Disadvantages
- **C:** Complications
- **P:** Prognosis

CONDITIONS

Adenomyosis

D: Diffuse or localized presence of endometrial tissue within the myometrium. If localized to one large area it is known as an adenomyoma.

A: Unknown. ? Direct invasion by overlying endometrium. ? Metaplastic change of tissue surrounding myometrial vessels giving rise to endometrial stroma and glandular tissue. ? Migration of decidua (the endometrium becomes deciduous during pregnancy) with uterine contractions during labour.

A/R: Endometriosis, fibroids, long period of secondary subfertility, multiparity, ↑ age.

E: Unknown, underestimated as diagnosis is based on histopathology. Occurs in 20–40 % of hysterectomy specimens.

H: 30 % asymptomatic.
Menstrual problems: menorrhagia, dysmenorrhoea (premenstrual and menstrual, peaking in later stages), ↑ frequency, spotting. **Others:** deep dyspareunia. Subfertility.
Symptoms regress after menopause as lesions are oestrogen dependent.

E: **Bimanual:** uterus (?↑ size, premenstrual and menstrual tenderness).

P: **Macro:** diffuse enlargement of uterus, thickened walls (posterior > anterior), absence of pseudocapsule formation around lesions (as seen in fibroids).
Micro: endometrial tissue within myometrium (stroma > glandular tissue). Proliferative cyclical variations seen in more mature tissue.

I: **Diagnostic:** transvaginal USS or MRI, hysteroscopy and histology of endometrial biopsy.
Exclusion of other causes: *Bloods*: FBC (↓ Hb), clotting screen. *Urine*: β-hCG (exclude pregnancy). *Others*: cervical smear (exclude cancer), laparoscopy (exclude endometriosis).

M: Treat symptomatic cases only.
Medical:
1 antifibrinolytics (tranexamic acid);
2 NSAIDs (mefenamic acid—helps with pain and bleeding);
3 GnRH agonists (buserelin);
4 IUS (Mirena);
5 COC;
6 progesterone (e.g. norethisterone).
Surgical (if medical treatment unsuccessful): abdominal hysterectomy with preservation of ovaries. If adenomyoma present can use local excision of lesion.

C: Anaemia. Malignant change to adenocarcinoma (rare).

P: Adenomyosis rarely responds to hormonal therapy, so most women will eventually require a hysterectomy to control symptoms.

Amenorrhoea

D: Absence of menstruation. Primary amenorrhoea is failure to establish menstruation. Secondary amenorrhoea is absence of menstruation for ≥ 6 consecutive months in a woman who has previously established regular menses.

A: Primary (5 %):
1 *Constitutional delay*: most common cause of primary.
2 *Obstructive*: imperforate hymen, transverse vaginal septum, absent or non-functioning uterus.
3 *Hormonal*: Kallmann's syndrome, weight loss, hyperprolactinoma.
4 *Congenital*: Androgen insensitivity syndrome, Turner's syndrome, gonadal agenesis, CAH.
5 *Others*: ovarian failure (e.g. chemotherapy/radiotherapy), pituitary tumour.

Secondary (95 %):
1 *Pregnancy*: most common cause of secondary amenorrhoea and should always be considered first.
2 *Ovary* (60 % of pathological causes): PCOS (35 %), premature ovarian failure (25 %).
3 *Pituitary* (20 %): hyperprolactinoma (17 %), hypopituitarism, Sheehan's syndrome, trauma, tumour, post OCP insensitivity.
4 *Hypothalamus*: hypothalamic hypogonadism (extreme exercise, ↓ weight, e.g. anorexia nervosa, idiopathic or chronic illness may result in thalamic suppression).
5 *Uterus* (rare): Asherman's syndrome, tuberculous endometritis.
6 *Others*: endocrine (thyroid disease, Cushing's).

A/R: n/a.

E: Not uncommon.

H: Assess LMP, menarche, previous menstrual history, contraception now and previously, possibility of pregnancy, weight loss, exercise, hirsuitism, galactorrhoea, vision, thyroid symptoms, climacteric symptoms and last smear date.

E: May be unremarkable.
Primary: delayed puberty, signs of underlying causes, e.g. imperforate hymen.
Secondary: signs of underlying cause, e.g. low weight, signs of PCOS.

P: n/a.

I: Tailor according to history and examination. Consider: *Bloods*: FSH, LH estradiol, androgens, prolactin, TFTs, SHBG. *Urine*: β-hCG (exclude pregnancy). *Others*: Anterior pituitary function tests, pelvic USS, visual fields, X-ray pituitary fossa. In primary amenorrhoea chromosomal studies may be indicated.

M: Depends on underlying cause.

C: Long-standing amenorrhoea can lead to osteoporosis and menopausal symptoms and signs.

P: Depends on underlying cause.

Amniotic fluid embolism

D: The presence of amniotic fluid in the maternal circulation.

A: Appears to be a combination of increased amniotic fluid pressure and a defect near the placental site allowing access into the maternal circulation.

A/R: Multiparity, uterine hyperstimulation (oxytocin use), rapid labour, caesarean section, increased maternal age.

E: 1 in 80 000 pregnancies.

H: Sudden-onset dyspnoea, often pink frothy sputum. ? Loss of consciousness.

E: **Output failure:** tachycardia, hypotension, cold sweaty peripheries, cyanosis, raised JVP.
Cardiac arrest: pulseless, no respiratory effort.
Seizures.
Coagulation failure: petechial skin haemorrhage, bleeding at puncture sites.

P: Poorly understood (lack of human data). Recently established register for all cases.
Amniotic fluid thought to cause severe transient pulmonary artery spasm and ↑ pulmonary arterial pressure, with resultant hypoxia leading to myocardial and pulmonary capillary damage and left ventricular failure. Activation of coagulation cascade → leakage of intravascular fluid to intraalveolar and interstitial spaces.

I: *Bloods*: FBC, U&E, LFT, ABG, cross-match 6 units.

M: CPR (if required).
High flow oxygen ± intubation, IPPV.
Insert two large-bore cannulae, take blood sample, IV fluids (crystalloid/colloid).
Use cross-matched blood if needed.
Fresh frozen plasma (if fibrinogen low).
Consider delivery.
Transfer to ITU.
Treat ARDS/ARF.

C: Cardiorespiratory arrest, DIC, left ventricular failure, haemorrhage, pulmonary oedema, ARDS, ARF, uterine atony, convulsions.

P: 80 % maternal mortality.

Anaemia in pregnancy

D: Haemoglobin level < 10.4 g/dL.

A: Most common cause is iron deficiency, but all other causes of anaemia must be considered.
Microcytic: iron deficiency, thalassaemia.
Macrocytic: *Megaloblastic:* folate/B_{12} deficiency (unlikely to be B_{12} deficiency as severe deficiency causes infertility). *Non-megaloblastic:* excessive alcohol, hypothyroidism, pregnancy itself, haemolysis.
Normocytic: haemorrhage (APH, PPH), haemolysis, anaemia of chronic disease, hydraemia of pregnancy (caused by dilution).

A/R: **Iron deficiency:** vegetarian/vegan diet, multiparity, previous menorrhagia.
Thalassaemia: family history, Mediterranean/Asian origin.
Folate deficiency: drugs (e.g. anticonvulsants), small bowel disease, malnutrition, haemolysis (e.g. sickle cell anaemia), malaria (in Africa).

E: Depends on population. ↑ Incidence seen in areas of ethnic minority (because of poor diet and ↑ incidence of haemoglobinopathies).

H: Asymptomatic (common), fatigue, dyspnoea, palpitations.

E: **General:** pallor, pale mucous membranes, ↑ capillary refill time, oedema. Signs of underlying cause may be present, e.g. mild jaundice in haemolysis.

P: ↓ Hb level is normal in pregnancy (a slight ↓ is associated with ↑ weight and well-being of fetus) as plasma volume expands at a greater rate than red cell volume causing dilution (especially with multiple pregnancy). Iron deficiency is more common in pregnancy as a result of ↑ iron demands secondary to ↑ red cell mass, new tissue formation (e.g. myometrium) and fetal demands. Lactation also ↑ demand for iron, and is associated with a higher incidence of anaemia in the post-partum period.

I: **Initial:** FBC, peripheral blood film, and MCV.
If ↓ Hb and ↓ MCV: serum iron, ferritin and total iron-binding capacity (TIBC). If normal consider Hb electrophoresis (exclude thalassaemia).
If ↓ Hb, ↓ MCV: serum iron, ferritin, TIBC, B_{12}, folate and red cell folate (exclude mixed picture). Tailor further tests according to clinical presentation.
If ↓ Hb and ↑ MCV: serum B_{12}, folate and red cell folate. If normal consider TFTs, LFTs, etc.

M: Treat underlying cause.
Iron deficiency: for anaemia detected early and Hb > 6.5 give oral $FeSO_4$ 60 mg/day. If < 4 weeks to delivery, anaemia severe or compliance problems give intramuscular iron. Blood transfusion is reserved for extreme circumstances. Avoid iron in thalassaemia and sickle cell anaemia.
Folate deficiency: oral folic acid supplement.

C: ↑ Susceptibility to complications of haemorrhage, SE of iron therapy (constipation, nausea—less well-tolerated in first trimester). ↑ Maternal mortality (5 ×), IUGR and stillbirth (6 ×).

P: Iron deficiency responds well to treatment.

Androgen insensitivity syndrome

D: X-linked recessive condition resulting in failure of testosterone to cause normal masculinization in the male (46 XY karyotype) leading to female phenotype with absent uterus. Complete or partial, depending on the amount of receptor function.

A: Mutation (deletions, insertions and point mutations) of the androgen receptor (*AR*) gene on the long arm of the X chromosome causing loss of function (receptor loss/altered substrate-binding affinity). Sometimes ↓ activity of enzyme converting testosterone to dihydrotestosterone or the testosterone receptor missing—testosterone produced in normal amounts but receptor-mediated events do not occur.

A/R: Family history (e.g. infertile unmarried aunt); male genotype.

E: 1 in 20 400 live males.

H: Amenorrhoea; lack of pubic and axillary hair; ? abnormal external genitalia.

E: Female appearance and voice; lack of pubic and axillary hair.
Complete: female external genitalia with normal breast development (testosterone converted to estradiol), labia, clitoris, and vaginal introitus.
Partial: variable phenotype from mildly virilized female to mildly undervirilized male external genitalia; absent uterus; ? testes palpable in the abdomen or groin.

P: Histology of the testes: normal testicular structure, ↓ sperm numbers post puberty. Testes produce normal amounts of müllerian-inhibiting factor (MIF) which causes regression of müllerian duct therefore absent fallopian tubes, uterus, or an upper vagina. Variable anatomical deviations may occur, from clitoromegaly, without other external anomalies, to hypospadias.

I: **Karyotyping:** *Bloods*: testosterone ↑; negative progesterone challenge; can measure dihydrotestosterone, dihydroepiandrosterone (DHEA), androstenedione, and their precursors, 17-hydroxypregnenolone and 17-hydroxyprogesterone (eliminate error). Rule out pregnancy/other causes amenorrhoea. *USS*: absence of uterus, location of testes.

M: **Medical:** oestrogen replacement therapy after the development of secondary sexual characteristics and removal of gonads. Combination with progesterone controversial.
Surgical: removal of gonads after the development of secondary sexual characteristics; vaginal lengthening procedures. Cosmetic procedures for masculinized genitalia.
Other: psychological support. Parental genetic counselling (risk of recurrence). Support groups.

C: Testicular malignancy (therefore orchidectomy recommended); infertility; extreme psychological trauma; osteoporosis; symptoms of oestrogen deficiency.

P: Good provided that adequate care and support is available.

Asherman's syndrome

D: Presence of intrauterine adhesions, which partially or completely occlude the uterine cavity, following instrumentation or infection.

A: Damage to the endometrium involving the basal layer, which leads to fibrosis and adhesion formation.

A/R: Endometrial resection (diathermy/laser ablation); excessive curettage (following miscarriage, therapeutic abortion, post-partum haemorrhage); surgery (myomectomy, caesarean section); endometritis (especially tuberculous and schistosomiasis infection).

E: Up to 20 % prevalence following ERPC (includes mild cases).

H: Women may present with abnormal menstruation (secondary amenorrhoea or hypomenorrhoea). Previous uterine instrumentation/infection. Dysmenorrhoea.

E: No physical signs.

P: Intrauterine adhesions/synechiae. Varying degree of uterine cavity occlusion.

I: *Bloods*: weekly progesterone (ovulatory range does not correspond with menstruation). *Other*: progestogen challenge test (no menstruation occurs). Hysterosalpingogram. Hysteroscopy.

M: Insert a large IUCD *or* hysteroscopic adhesiolysis + IUCD (1 week), antibiotic coverage, high-dose oestrogen (21 days) and a progestogen (10 days) to induce endometrial proliferation.

C: Infertility. Pregnancy complications: premature rupture of membranes, preterm labour, fetal hypoxia and caesarean hysterectomy (if pregnancy occurs).

P: 50 % likelihood of subsequent infertility in more severe cases.

Atrophic vaginitis

D: Atrophy of the vagina and vulva with thinning of the epithelium.

A: ↓ In circulating oestrogen levels.

A/R: Prior to menarche, prolonged lactation, postmenopausal.

E: Postmenopausal women mostly affected. Common cause of postmenopausal bleeding.

H: Bloodstained, sometimes purulent, vaginal discharge. Vaginal dryness and dyspareunia. Superimposed infection with Gram-positive cocci or Gram-negative bacilli can worsen symptoms.

E: **Pelvic:** *Speculum*: thin pale inflamed vaginal wall with loss of rugal folds. Petechial haemorrhages and occasionally ecchymoses.

P: ↓ Stimulatory effects of oestrogen result in a loss of glycogen in the epithelial cells and a decrease in vaginal acidity, which results in ↑ risk of superimposed infection.

I: **Exclude malignancy:** cervical smear, HVS (exclude superimposed infection), USS (usually transvaginal, but transabdominal if vagina too tight. Endometrial thickness assessed), hysteroscopy.

M: Vaginal pH and epithelium must be restored.
Medical: 1 Dienestrol cream topically. Applied once a day at night for 1 week, followed by monthly application to prevent atrophy.
2 Systemic HRT in postmenopausal women.

C: Increased frequency of UTI resulting from atrophy of lower urinary tract, psychosexual problems resulting from dyspareunia, infection, side-effects from excessive absorption of topical oestrogen.

P: Treatment successful in majority of patients.

Bacterial vaginosis

D: An alteration in vaginal flora with excessive anaerobic bacteria, e.g. *Gardnerella vaginalis, Mycoplasma hominis.*

A: Ill-understood alteration in vaginal flora accompanied by reduced level of vaginal lactobacilli. Organisms naturally colonize the female tract—therefore thought to be a colonization rather than infection.

A/R: Smoking; multiple sexual partners; low socioeconomic status.

E: 15% prevalence in antenatal clinics.

H: Copious grey malodorous discharge; fishy odour exacerbated during menstruation/following intercourse (as a result of alkalinity); pain and pruritus uncommon.

E: Evidence of homogeneous grey discharge which adheres to vaginal wall. Little or no inflammation.

P: n/a

I: Bacterial vaginosis can only be diagnosed if three out of the four **Amsel criteria** are present.
1 Thick homogeneous white/grey discharge with offensive odour, which adheres to the vaginal walls.
2 Litmus—pH alkaline (> 4.5).
3 Fish amine test—positive; bacterial metabolites produce amines with distinct 'fishy' odour on addition of 10% KOH.
4 Microscopy—clue cells (vaginal epithelial cells with attached bacteria), NB: also ↓ lactobacilli.

M: Treatment unnecessary unless symptomatic/pregnant.
Medical: oral metronidazole, topical clindamycin (especially in first trimester).
Advice: avoid vaginal douching (alters vaginal acidity).

C: Associations shown with PROM, preterm labour, chorioamnionitis, cervical dysplasia.

P: Often recurs but should remain untreated unless pregnant or symptomatic.

Bartholinitis

D: Inflammation of Bartholin's gland(s) secondary to bacterial infection.

A: **Commensal flora:** staphylococcus, *Escherichia coli*, *Enterococcus faecalis*, *Mycoplasma hominis*.
Sexually transmitted: *Neisseria gonorrhoea*, *Chlamydia trachomatis*.

A/R: Damage to duct of Bartholin's gland (sexual trauma, surgery, episiotomy), immunocompromised, unprotected intercourse.

E: Most common bacterial infection of vulva affecting women of reproductive age. Occurs in 2% of women, and 25% of those with gonococcal infection.

H: Acute pain around introitus, difficulty in sitting down, superficial dyspareunia, lump around vagina, difficulty with tampon use.

E: **General:** tachycardia, pyrexia if systemic infection (rare).
Pelvic: palpable red tender fluctuant mass at posterior part of labia majora on fourchette. Usually unilateral. Oedema of surrounding tissue. Tender inguinal lymph nodes.

P: The pea-sized Bartholin's glands are located laterally to and outside the hymen within the vestibular bulbs. They each connect to the posterior part of the vestibule by a small narrow duct 1–2 cm long, which is prone to infection as a result of its narrow nature. The glands function to produce mucus during coitus. Chronic occlusion of the duct may result in a Bartholin's cyst, which can be large, and is either lined by the transitional epithelium of the normal duct or by squamous metaplasia.

I: *Bloods*: FBC (WCC—exclude systemic infection). *Others*: urethral and endocervical swab (to diagnose gonococcal infection if present), culture of pus from abscess (for antibiotic sensitivity).

M: **Medical:** analgesia, broad-spectrum antibiotics until sensitivity known.
Surgical: if abscess or cyst, treat by marsupialization (abscess wall incised and vaginal and walls of abscess are stitched open. Drain may be used for 1–2 days). Biopsy of gland for histology. In older women, gland may be removed to exclude rare possibility of malignancy.

C: **Acute bartholinitis:** abscess formation. **Chronic low-grade infection:** cyst formation as a result of occlusion of duct leading to retention of mucus products. Systemic infection (rare).

P: Recurrence rate low with marsupialization. Recurrence rate and incidence of cysts may be higher if other surgical procedures are used.

Benign ovarian mass

D: Includes 'chocolate' (endometrioma), dermoid, epithelial, functional cysts (follicular and luteal) and fibromas, and the rare sex cord tumours. (NB some of these may also be malignant.)

A: Unknown, probably oestrogen related. Dermoid cysts are congenital.

A/R: Erratic hormone levels (puberty, menopause), ↑ oestrogen levels (ovulation induction, obesity, PCOS) oestrogen exposure (early menarche, late menopause, nulliparity), ↑ age (except dermoid cyst), family history. Reduced risk: COC pill, pregnancy, multiparity.

E: One in three women at some point in life. Dermoid cyst most common in < 30 years, physiological are most common in reproductive years, others are most common after menopause.

H: Often asymptomatic.
Acute (as a result of torsion): sudden onset of severe colicky lower abdominal pain, syncope.
Chronic: abdominal swelling/discomfort, pressure symptoms (urinary/GI), menstrual irregularities (rare).

E: *Acute:* shock, fever, lower abdominal peritonism.
Chronic: Abdomen: distension, pelvic mass, ascites (Meigs' syndrome).
Bimanual: painless cystic or solid mass.

P: **Physiological (25 %):** *Follicular:* unruptured graafian follicle resulting from failed rupture of non-dominant follicle or failure of non-dominant to degenerate. Usually small (< 5 cm). Lined by granulosa cells. *Luteal:* usually unilateral, > 3 cm by definition. Lined by luteal cells.
Dermoid cyst (mature cystic teratoma): bilateral in 10 %, usually unilocular cyst < 15 cm. Derived from germ cells, therefore may contain ectodermal tissue (squamous epithelium, teeth, hair, sebaceous glands), endodermal tissue (thyroid, intestine) or mesodermal tissue (cartilage).
Epithelial: *Serous cystadenoma:* **most common epithelial tumour**, bilateral in 10 %. Thin-walled, uniloculated and filled with watery fluid. Lined by cuboidal epithelium. May contain psammoma bodies (calcified bodies). *Mucinous cystadenoma:* usually large, unilateral, multiloculated and filled with thick fluid. Lined by mucous secreting columnar cells. *Brenner:* rare small solid-looking tumour, bilateral in 15 %. Contains transitional epithelium (Walthard nests).
Sex cord: *Theca:* often produce oestrogen. *Fibroma:* hard, mobile and shiny white. *Granulosa:* usually malignant.
Chocolate cyst: occurs in endometriosis when endometrial tissue is present in ovary. The lesion becomes filled with altered blood ('melted chocolate' appearance).

I: *Acute: Bloods:* FBC, clotting, U&Es, cross-match. *Urine:* β-hCG.
Chronic: Bloods: FBC (Hb, WCC) ESR, CRP (PID), Ca 125 (ovarian cancer). *Urine:* β hCG (exclude pregnancy). *Others:* transvaginal/pelvic USS (diagnostic), paracentesis of ascites.

M: ↑ **Risk of malignancy** (e.g. USS appearance, Ca 125 levels, > 45 year): laparotomy or laparoscopy (avoid if malignancy possible), and BSO. Consider TAH. HRT following surgery. ↓ **Risk of malignancy:** observe if < 10 cm. If no resolution after 8 weeks, or cyst > 10 cm, laparoscopy (preferably) or laparotomy and cystectomy.

C: **All:** Accident (rupture, torsion, haemorrhage), subfertility, malignancy change. **Fibroma:** Meigs' syndrome (ascites and pleural effusion—rare). **Mucinous cystadenoma:** pseudomyxoma peritonei (abdominal cavity filled

Benign ovarian mass continued

with gelatinous material). **Dermoid cyst**: hyperthyroidism (if thyroid tissue present).

P: Surgery usually curative.

β-Haemolytic streptococcus—Groups A and B

D: Upper genital tract infection/neonatal infection caused by β-haemolytic streptococcus groups A (*Streptococcus pyogenes*) or B (*Streptococcus agalactiae*).

A: Group A: transmission by aerosol/direct skin contact (from birth attendant).
Group B: gut commensal commonly colonizes vagina during pregnancy. *Uterine infection/chorioamnionitis*: ascending infection following rupture of membranes. *Puerperal sepsis*: ascending infection and bacterial spread though placental site/genital tract lacerations. *Neonatal infection (only B)*: during passage through birth canal.

A/R: Low socioeconomic status, low parity.
Puerperal sepsis: caesarean section, PROM, prolonged labour, instrumental delivery, retained products of conception.
Neonatal infection: premature labour, PROM, IUGR, birth asphyxia.

E: Group A: < 1 % genital tract infection during pregnancy.
Group B: 5–20 % of women. *Neonatal infection*: 0.5–1 % of babies born through colonized birth canal. *Puerperal sepsis*: 3 % of colonized women.

H: Vaginal colonization: often asymptomatic.
Puerperal sepsis: malaise, headache, fever, rigors, abdominal discomfort, backache, vaginal bleeding, vomiting, diarrhoea, offensive lochia.
Neonatal infection: fever, irritable, poor feeding, vomiting/asymptomatic.

E: Puerperal sepsis: pyrexia, tachycardia, large boggy tender uterus, signs of peritonism.
Neonatal infection: *Early onset* (within hours): irritability, tachypnoea, apnoea, convulsions, signs of respiratory distress, circulatory collapse, DIC. *Late onset* (1–4 weeks): asymptomatic, signs of meningitis.

P: Puerperal sepsis: infection of uterus, bacteraemia.
Neonatal infection: bacteraemia, bacterial infection of lungs meninges/other organs.

I: *Bloods* (mother and neonate): FBC, U&E, culture (severe infection). *Other*: vaginal swab + culture (if complicated pregnancy, previous premature labour, prolonged rupture of membranes); amniotic fluid sample and culture (PROM).

M: Group A identified: isolate patient, IV benzyl penicillin/oral amoxicillin (milder infection).
Group B identified: immediate delivery (if PROM), intrapartum/sepsis treatment IV ampicillin (also prophylactic use in PROM, prolonged rupture of membranes) and perinatal penicillin given to neonate (until culture results available).
Neonatal infection: IV penicillin and aminoglycoside, treat complications.

C: Vaginal colonization: upper genital tract infection, preterm labour, PROM, associated with miscarriage, neonatal infection.
Puerperal sepsis: peritonitis, septicaemic shock, death.
Neonatal infection: respiratory distress syndrome, septicaemia, meningitis, death.

P: Neonatal infection: up to 80 % mortality.
Puerperal sepsis: low mortality in the UK; however, higher worldwide.

Candida albicans infection of the genital tract

D: Overgrowth of naturally occurring *Candida albicans* in the vulva and/or vagina.

A: *Candida* proliferation occurs when the pH within the vagina is more alkaline.

A/R: Immunocompromised, pregnancy, sexually active (but is not an STI), diabetes mellitus, broad-spectrum antibiotic therapy, wearing of nylon underwear and tights.

E: Very common. Experienced by >90 % women at some point in life.

H: Pruritus vulvae, soreness, superficial dyspareunia, 'cottage cheese'-like non-offensive discharge.

E: **Pelvic:** *Inspection*: vaginal discharge, vaginal fissures and erythematous indurated vulva. White plaques may be seen on vulva and vaginal wall which may bleed when removed.

A: A yeast which infects the epitheloid cells where it develops spores and pseudohyphae. May lie dormant within cells until conditions encourage growth, e.g. ↑ vaginal pH.
Microscopy: budding yeasts, spores and pseudohyphae. Cultured on Sabouraud's medium.

I: HVS for microscopy and culture.

M: **Advice:** cotton underwear, wiping anus front to back, etc.
Medical: 500 mg single dose clotrimazole vaginal pessary ± topical 10 % clotrimazole cream (e.g. Canesten) or 150 mg oral fluconazole (e.g. Diflucan) if not pregnant. Treat the partner if recurrent infections.
Recurrent attacks: consider prophylactic treatment, e.g. weekly pessary or oral fluconazole (150 mg).

C: Distress and disruption to social and sexual life (recurrent attacks)

P: With the above management 85 % are cured. 5–15 % of women have recurrent attacks which is usually a result of relapse of initial infection.

Carcinoma of the cervix

D: Malignant change in the cervical epithelium.

A: Unknown; however, see AR; HPV 16 and 18 implicated because of ability to cause tumorigenesis in immunocompromised animals. HPV oncogenes cause tumour growth by binding to the tumour suppressor protein p53.

A/R: Smoking; multiple sexual partners; age at first intercourse; lower socio-economic status; HIV.

E: Most common around 45–50 years.

H: Intermenstrual vaginal bleeding; postmenopausal bleeding; post-coital bleeding; sometimes offensive/bloodstained discharge.
Late symptoms: symptoms from metastasis; lower limb oedema; pelvic/sciatic pain; difficulty voiding (obstruction); incontinence (fistula); non-specific (e.g. weight loss).

E: Speculum and VE: friable exophytic (grow outwards) growths, indurated or ulcerated cervix; examination may be normal if malignancy develops within the endocervical canal or in early stages of disease.
Late: pelvic/rectal/abdominal mass.

P: Squamous cell carcinoma (ectocervical) 90 %; adenocarcinoma (endocervical) 10 %.

Stage Ia   Microinvasion.
Stage Ib   Confined to cervix.
Stage IIa Extends to upper vagina.
Stage IIb Extends to parametrium.
Stage IIIa Extends to lower vagina.
Stage IIIb Reaches pelvic wall/? ureteric obstruction.
Stage IVa Extends to bladder/rectum.
Stage IVb Haematogenous spread (e.g. bowel/lungs).

I: Repeat smear or → colposcopy with biopsy; staging cystoscopy, sigmoidoscopy, colposcopy with biopsy; CXR (secondaries); IVU if genitourinary obstruction. *Bloods:* Hb (anaemia); U&E (if obstruction); LFT (liver metastases uncommon but may occur in advanced disease).

M: **Surgery:** *Stage Ia*: cone biopsy, hysterectomy if appropriate. *Stages Ib–IIa*: radical hysterectomy (Wertheim), bilateral pelvic lymphadenectomy.
Radiotherapy: fractionated external radiation and intracervical and intravaginal caesium if above Stage IIb; unsuitable for surgery (e.g. elderly); node positive; large tumours.
Chemotherapy: advanced disease.
Chemoradiation: 5 fluorouracil with cisplastin/carboplatin.
Follow-up: initially 3-monthly progressing to 6-monthly for 5 years. Yearly smears.

C: Spread to uterus, upper vagina, rectum, bladder, parametrium. Lymphatic spread to pelvic and para-aortic nodes. Effects of radiotherapy (necrosis, fibrosis, stenosis, inflammation, fistulae). Genitourinary obstruction; bladder and rectal fistulae formation.

P: May be related principally to tumour size at diagnosis; also spread and recurrence; adenocarcinoma worse prognosis.

Carcinoma of endometrium

D: Malignancy of endometrial tissue.

A: Unknown.

A/R: Unopposed oestrogen stimulation of endometrium.
Exogenous: oestrogen-only HRT, tamoxifen.
Endogenous: nulliparity, early menarche, late menopause, PCOS, oestrogen-producing ovarian tumours (granulosa/theca), obesity (? aromatization of fat-derived peripheral androgens).
Others: carbohydrate intolerance, family history of bowel, ovarian or endometrial cancer (Lynch II syndrome/Hereditary non-polyposis colon cancer syndrome) hypertension. ↓ Risk with COC pill or HRT.

E: Second most common cancer of genital tract after ovarian cancer. In UK, 5100 cases per year. Lifetime risk ~1%. Peak incidence ~60 years (5% <40 years).

H: Postmenopausal bleeding, menorrhagia (if premenopausal), watery vaginal discharge, lower abdominal pain.

E: Usually normal.
General: signs of malignancy (anaemia, cachexia).
Pelvic: enlarged groin lymph nodes.
Bimanual: uterus: enlargement and irregular softening.

P: **Macro:** lesions seen as raised rough areas on hysteroscopy. Spread occurs locally and lymphatically (haematological spread occurs late). *Stage I*: confined to uterus. a, In endometrium; b, invasion < 1/2 myometrial thickness; c, > 1/2 myometrial thickness. *Stage II*: confined to uterus and cervix. a, Endocervical gland involvement; b, stromal involvement. *Stage III*: beyond uterus, confined to pelvis. *Stage IV*: beyond pelvis. a, Bowel or bladder; b, distant metastases.
Micro: 80% adenocarcinoma (resembles proliferative phase endometrium); 20% adenosquamous (malignant glandular and squamous tissue) or other, e.g. clear cell carcinoma. Atypical hyperplasia of endometrium may precede cancer.

I: **Diagnostic:** USS (exclude endometrial cancer if endometrium <4mm. Also exclude ovarian pathology), hysteroscopy and endometrial biopsy (diagnostic), cervical smear (exclude cervical cancer), CXR (metastatic spread).
Bloods: FBC (↓ Hb). *Urine:* β-hCG (if premenopausal, exclude pregnancy), haematuria, malignant cells (metastatic spread).
Assess fitness for surgery: *Bloods:* FBC (↓ Hb), U&E, clotting, LFT, crossmatch 4 units; CXR, ECG.

M: Psychological support and counselling.
Stage I and II: Laparotomy with TAH, BSO and removal of upper part of vagina. *Follow-up*: vaginal vault radiotherapy to selected women (e.g. not Stage Ia) to ↓ risk of recurrence in vaginal vault. External beam radiotherapy to high-risk patients for LN involvement (deep myometrial involvement, poor differentiation, cervical stroma involvement).
Stage III and IV: multidisciplinary care. *Medical:* radiotherapy, chemotherapy, progesterone therapy. Palliative care if treatment fails.

C: Metastatic spread resulting in bowel obstruction and urinary symptoms. Psychological effects. Recurrence. Complications from treatment.

P: 65% overall 5-year survival rate, depends on stage (Stage I, 75%; Stage IV, 10%), differentiation, tumour type (adenocarcinoma has worse prognosis than adenosquamous), and LN involvement.

Carcinoma of ovary

D: Malignant tumour arising from ovarian epithelial cells.

A: Malignant change of benign tumour/premalignant phase not recognized. 5–10 % attributed to hereditary factors: *BRCA 1* (Chromosome 17—risk of developing ovarian ca $\leq$ 45%), *BRCA 2* (Chromosome 13—↑ risk of developing ovarian ca by 20%), mismatch repair genes.

A/R: **Higher number of ovulations:** nulliparity, early menarche, late menopause, prolonged ovulation induction, family history, advanced age.
Protective: COC pill, pregnancy, lactation.

E: Most common gynaecological malignancy: 5000 new cases per year (UK). Peak incidence: 50–70 years of age.

H: Asymptomatic (initially), abdominal pain, swelling/mass, pressure symptoms: urinary frequency/retention, constipation, abnormal menses (rare), weight loss, malaise, dyspepsia, GI/breast symptoms (metastases).

E: Enlarged abdomen, palpable abdominal/pelvic mass, ascites, cachexia.

P: **Stage I** Disease confined to ovaries.
Stage II Disease extends into pelvis.
Stage III Disease spread but confined to abdomen.
Stage IV Distant metastases or spread to liver.
Histology: serous papillary cystadenocarcinoma (fluid-filled cystic components), most common; mucinous adenocarcinoma (mucin-filled cysts); endometroid carcinoma (resembles endometrial adenocarcinoma); clear cell carcinoma (cells have clear cytoplasm); Brenner tumour (transitional epithelium); borderline tumour (any of the above histology, low malignant potential).

I: *Bloods*: FBC, U&E, LFT, Ca 125 (↑ in >80% of patients, therefore tumour marker, treatment response), AFP, β-hCG, estradiol (sex cord/stromal tumour suspected). *Imaging*: ultrasound pelvis ± CT/MRI. *Other*: laparoscopy/laparotomy (diagnostic staging and treatment).

M: Counsel patient, multidisciplinary management. Follow-up ∼ 5 years.
Curative: *Surgery*: TAH, BSO, infracolic omentectomy, inspection and sampling of lymph nodes, removal of other macroscopic disease if possible (Stage III and IV), consider conservative surgery (young nulliparous women). *Chemotherapy*: (Stages II–IV, ? Ic) carboplatin/cisplatin + Taxol. *Radioimmunotherapy*: still experimental.
Palliative: (incurable disease) adequate analgesia (step up as needed), antiemetics, radiotherapy (for vaginal bleeding), paracentesis (ascites), surgery.

C: Torsion, rupture, haemorrhage, impaction, metastatic spread (NB peritoneal seeding), small bowel obstruction, complications of treatment, death.

P: Stage-dependant 5-year survival (epithelial tumours):
Stage I   60–70 %
Stage II   30 %
Stage III 10 %
Stage IV   5 %.

Carcinoma of the vulva

- **D:** Malignancy of the vulva. Includes SCC, BCC, VC, MM and other rarer ones.
- **A:** Unknown. Two current hypotheses:
  1. *de novo* (seen in elderly patients in association with other diseases);
  2. associated with progression of VIN (HPV associated—seen in younger women).
- **A/R:**
  1. Associated with *de novo*. ↑ Age, lichen sclerosus, diabetes, hypertension, obesity, schistosomiasis, lymphogranuloma venereum and squamous hyperplasia.
  2. VIN, smoking.
- **E:** 1 in 100 000 women per year. 1 in 3 patients > 70 years. Accounts for 400 deaths per year.
- **H:** Pruritus vulvae, lump or ulcer-like lesion, bleeding. Occasionally offensive purulent discharge.
- **E:** **Pelvic inspection:** *SCC*: nodule/ulcer, usually on labia majora or clitoris. Bloodstained discharge with offensive odour. Groin lymphadenopathy (hard, immobile). *BCC*: ulcerated nodule, usually on labia. *VC*: wart-like lesion. *MM:* highly pigmented lesion.
- **P:** 80 % are SCC which are well differentiated with keratinization and have a relatively high rate (∼10 %) of metastases to local lymph nodes. Of the remaining 20 %, the most common types are BCC, VC and MM. BCC and VC rarely metastasize but MM has a high rate of metastasis. The rarer cancers include Paget's disease, other types of adenocarcinoma, sarcoma and metastatic tumours. Staged according to International Federation of Gynaecology and Obstetrics (FIGO) criteria:
  Stage Ia Tumour < 2.0 cm with < 1 mm of dermal invasion. No lymphatic involvement and node negative.
  Stage Ib As above but with > 1 mm of dermal invasion.
  Stage II Tumour > 2.0 cm confined to vulva or perineum with no node involvement.
  Stage III Tumour any size with spread to lower urethra ± vagina, anus unilateral groin node involvement.
  Stage IVa Tumour of any size invading any of upper urethra, bladder mucosa, rectal mucosa, pelvic bone or bilateral groin nodes.
  Stage IVb Distant metastases.
- **I:** **Diagnostic:** biopsy of lesion and histology. Sentinal node biospy. Cervical smear (exclude CIN in those associated with VIN).
  Assess fitness for surgery: *Bloods*: FBC, U&E, CXR, ECG.
- **M:** **Surgery:** triple incision vulvectomy and bilateral node dissection. Smaller lateral (> 2 cm from midline) lesions can be treated with WLE and unilateral node dissection.
  Medical: radiotherapy (RT) if LN involvement. Chemotherapy is being used increasingly in conjunction with radiotherapy.
- **C:** Psychological trauma.
  Tumour: voiding difficulties, haemorrhage from nodal involvement. Secondary infection of lesion.
  Surgery: haemorrhage, TED, infection, etc. Lymphoedema of leg as a result of node dissection. (In the future lymphatic mapping and sentinel node biopsy will reduce the need for node dissection and therefore complications resulting from it.)
  RT: erythema, desquamation, pubic symphysis and femoral head necrosis, fistula formation.

Carcinoma of the vulva continued

P: Depends on stage and type, e.g. SCC has a 90 % 5-year survival for Stage I, 40 % for Stage III. Malignant melanomas and adenocarcinomas have a very poor prognosis with 5 % 5-year survival.

Cardiac disease in pregnancy

D: Pre-existing cardiac disease in a pregnant woman.

A: Disorders including PDA, ASD, VSD, coarctation, Fallot's tetralogy, aortic stenosis, Eisenmenger's syndrome, acquired valvular defects (e.g. post-rheumatic fever, ischaemia etc.).

A/R: As for cardiac disease.

E: 0.5–2 % of pregnancies.

H: Previous history of cardiac disease; ≥ 1 of following ↑ SOB; paroxysmal nocturnal dyspnoea; ↓ exercise tolerance; palpitations; fatigue; ↓ fetal movements.

E: CVS: check—pulse; BP; JVP; oedema; basal crepitations; murmurs (NB ejection systolic common in pregnancy).
Abdomen: ↓ fundal height.

P: 40 % increase in blood volume during pregnancy (returns to normal by 4 weeks post-partum) → may increase strain in cardiac disease. Cardiac output rises from 3–5 L/min to 6–7.5 L/min at 36 weeks (because of reduced peripheral resistance) → may not be achieved with cardiac disease.

I: Pulse oximetry. *Bloods*: Hb.
Echocardiography (extent of impairment).
Cardiac anomaly scan ~ 22 weeks.
Screen for IUGR (especially right → left shunts as decreases PO_2).

M: Combined cardiology/obstetric hospital-based tertiary care.
Watch for: pre-eclampsia, multiple pregnancy, UTI/chest infections, subacute bacterial endocarditis, AF, anaemia (all ↑ cardiac strain). Anticoagulate with heparin instead of warfarin in valvular disease (↓ teratogenicity).
Marfan's and Eisenmenger's: admit from second trimester. *Signs of cardiac failure*: admit and consult cardiologist (re digoxin and diuretic therapy).
Labour: confer with anaesthetist prior to delivery; antibiotic prophylaxis prior to delivery with valvular disease; avoid ergometrine during delivery (→ hypertension); semi sitting position (↓ risk cardiac failure as ↑ venous return post labour); aim for vaginal delivery with short second stage (CS → ↑ risks); good pain relief (↓ pain-related stress)—epidural if avoid hypotension.
Advice: counsel with respect to risks and care. Prenatal counselling for future pregnancies.

C: **Maternal:** possible cardiac failure post-partum (post contractional increases in cardiac volume); risk of shunt reversal; mortality.
Fetal: ↑ risk fetal malformations; IUGR; preterm labour.

P: Cardiac failure most likely within 24 h delivery; 60 % deaths post delivery. Mortality most likely in conditions which prevent increases in cardiac output, e.g. pulmonary hypertension and mitral stenosis; greatest risk with Eisenmenger's—30 % risk mortality. Remains a significant contributor to maternal mortality in the UK.

Cervical ectopy (erosion) and eversion (ectropion)

D: Ectopy (erosion): extension of the columnar epithelium of the endocervical canal on to the ectocervix.
Eversion: as above, but with different cause and appearance.

A: Ectopy: ↑ oestrogen levels.
Eversion: minor, bilateral lacerations to the cervix during childbirth.

A/R: Ectopy: puberty, COC pill, pregnancy, diethystilbestrol exposure *in utero*.
Eversion: trauma during delivery, e.g. instrumental intervention, large baby (> 4.0 kg).

E: Unknown as most cases asymptomatic. Ectopy is a normal finding in young women—5 % have a large area with extension in to the anterior and posterior fornices.

H: Asymptomatic, vaginal discharge (clear, non-offensive, non-itchy), post-coital bleeding.

E: Cusco speculum: *Ectopy*: regular, red, 'velvety' area around external os.
Eversion: irregular, red, 'velvety' area around external os.

P: The point at which the columnar epithelium of the endocervical canal meets the squamous epithelium of the ectocervix is called the squamocolumnar junction. Increased oestrogen levels results in expansions of cervical ground substance in the stroma leading to swelling and eversion by pouting. Following trauma during childbirth, the endocervical epithelium extends outwards around the damaged area. This is probably because of the influence of local substances, e.g. cytokines, promoting proliferation and hyperplasia.

I: HVS (exclude infection), cervical smear (exclude malignancy), colposcopy (exclude malignancy).

M: Reassure that condition is benign. If symptomatic consider Aci-Jel to lower vaginal pH and increase metaplasia of columnar epithelium to squamous epithelium. If this fails consider cryotherapy or diathermy.

C: Chronic cervicitis (columnar epithelium less resistant to infection). Squamous metaplasia of columnar epithelium → nabothian cysts.

P: n/a

Cervical intraepithelial neoplasia

D: The presence of premalignant cellular atypia within the squamous epithelium of the cervix.

A: Exact aetiology unknown. HPV (types 16 and 18) thought to be involved (implicated in the development of dysplasia).

A/R: Multiple sexual partners/partner with multiple previous partners. Early age of first coitus. Herpes simplex virus (type 2). Smoking. Immunosuppression. Lower socioeconomic status.

E: Peak incidence 20–30 years of age.

H: Commonly asymptomatic.

E: Generally no physical signs.

P: Dysplastic epithelial changes (↑ nuclear : cytoplasmic ratio)—↑ nuclear size, abnormal nuclear shape (poikilocytosis), increased nuclear density (koilocytosis), ↓ cytoplasm.
  CIN I   Mild dysplasia confined to lower third of the epithelium.
  CIN II Moderate dysplasia affecting two-thirds of the epithelial thickness.
  CIN III Severe dysplasia, carcinoma *in situ*.

I: Cervical smear (detection through cytological screening), colposcopy + biopsy (identify lesion).

M: CIN I: observe.
  CIN II or III: → LLETZ (diathermy)/laser treatment (small lesion)/cryotherapy/cone biopsy (glandular lesion/extension into cervical canal) + histology. Hysterectomy (CIN III + family complete).
  Follow-up: dependent on extent of disease and unit. Yearly smears for 5 years before re-entering normal screening programmes.

C: Carcinoma *in situ*, cervical carcinoma, psychological morbidity.

P: CIN I: 25 % progression to higher stages, 50 % regression (2 years).
  CIN III: 14–70 % estimated progression to carcinoma.

Cervicitis

D: Infection and inflammation of the cervix.

A: Caused by *Chlamydia* (~50%), gonococcus, papilloma virus, herpes virus. Chronic cervicitis often caused by mixed flora including *Trichomonas*, *Candida*, *Gardnerella*.

A/R: ↑ Number sexual partners; ↓ use of barrier contraceptive methods.

E: As for causative factor.

H: Acute: often asymptomatic. Vaginal discharge, may be purulent.
Chronic: persistent discharge; pelvic pain; dyspareunia; symptoms of urethral irritation.

E: Speculum: red, inflamed cervix; friable; evidence of discharge; chronic—enlarged, irregular cervix; ? retention cysts of cervical glands (nabothian follicles).
Bimanual: in chronic cervicitis ? cervix enlarged, hard and irregular (possible confusion with carcinoma).

P: Chronic cervicitis may → heavy lymphocytic and plasma cell infiltrate.

I: Bacteriology: cervical and high vaginal swabs.
Cervical cytology: refer for **colposcopy** if clinically suspicious.

M: Acute: antibacterial therapy targeted at infective agent.
Chronic: consider Aci-Jel (glacial acetic acid preparation) to ↓ vaginal pH and ↑ metaplasia columnar to squamous epithelium. Cauterization or cryotherapy to destroy inflamed columnar epithelium.
Follow-up to ensure eradication.

C: May obscure neoplasia on pap smear; acute may progress to chronic; ascending infection (especially during childbirth/cervical dilation); infertility; chronic pain; cervical stenosis or secondary haemorrhage from cauterization.

P: Acute: often successfully treated but may progress to chronic.
Chronic: subject to complications as mentioned above.

Chlamydia infection of the female genital tract

D: An STI caused by *Chlamydia trachomatis*.

A: Sexual intercourse with infected partner, 50 % transmission rate.

A/R: ↑ Number of partners, ↓ risk with use of barrier methods of contraception.

E: Currently most common STI in UK. Accounts for 50 % of cases of PID. Estimated 0.5–15 % of females infected, depending on population.

H: Can present with acute infection, acute or chronic PID. *Acute infection*: asymptomatic in ∼60 %. Vulval irritation, superficial dyspareunia, dysuria and frequency, vaginal discharge. *PID*: (see p. 57).

E: Acute infection: *Pelvic inspection*: copious mucous vaginal discharge, pain, induration. *Speculum*: cervicitis.
PID: (see p. 57).

P: Intracellular Gram-positive bacterium which has viral and bacterial characteristics. Several serovars; B–K cause infection described above and L1, L2 and L3 cause lymphogranuloma venereum (rare in UK). Consists of an infectious part (elementary body) and intracellular part (reticulate body). Elementary body attaches to epithelial cells of urethra, cervix, uterine tube and conjunctiva and is taken into cell. Reticulate body then replicates by binary fission forming intracellular inclusions. Cell then bursts releasing infectious elementary bodies. Diagnosis follows cell culture (required as intracellular organism) and ELISA or PCR.

I: Not yet part of national screening programme but, due to increases in incidence, it is likely to become part of one in future.
Acute infection: endocervical swab (culture and ELISA), first void urine (PCR or LCR). STI screen: HVS (TV, BV, *Candida*, gonorrhoea), blood sample (HIV, syphilis, hepatitis B).
Acute PID: FBC (↑ WCC), ESR, CRP, U&E.
Chronic PID: laparoscopy, hysterosalpingogram, dye test (tubal patency).

M: Acute infection: doxycycline 200 mg stat, then 100 mg/day for 1 week. Erythromycin for 1 week if systemic infection or azithromycin 1 g single dose. Repeat swab in 4 weeks (swabs may remain positive for up to 4 weeks) to ensure clearance.
Advice: avoid intercourse for 2 weeks. Contact tracing. PID: (see p. 57).

C: Ascending infection: acute/chronic PID (abscess, peritonitis, infertility, ectopic pregnancy, chronic pelvic pain) miscarriage, premature labour, Reiter's syndrome (characterized by arthritis, mucosal ulceration and conjunctivitis. Rare in women), Fitz-Hugh–Curtis syndrome (perihepatitis characterized by pyrexia, RUQ pain, guarding, abnormal LFT), conjunctivitis.
Neonate: ophthalmitis, pneumonia.

P: Acute PID results in tubal blockage in 15 % of cases following first episode, 40 % following second episode and 75 % following third episode. Early antibiotic therapy before tissue damage has occurred can be curative. Reversal of tubal damage may be impossible although new techniques of salpingoplasty may be of use. IVF for tubal infertility may be required.

Chronic hypertension in pregnancy

D: Hypertension (diastolic BP ≥ 90 mmHg on ≥ 2 occasions *or* diastolic BP ≥ 110 mmHg on 1 occasion) that is either present **prior** to conception, found at booking before 20 weeks' gestation or persists after pregnancy.

A: > 90 % essential. Remainder secondary to: *endocrine* (Cushing's, Conn's, phaeochromocytoma, CAH, acromegaly); *renal* (renal artery stenosis, chronic renal disease, e.g. chronic pyelonephritis); *vascular* (coarctation of aorta, collagen disorder of vessels).

A/R: ↑ Age, ethnicity (Afro-Caribbean), obesity, smoking, diabetes, family history, hypertension while taking COC pill, high salt intake.

E: 5 % (excluding pre-eclampsia and pregnancy induced hypertension) of pregnant women.

H: Asymptomatic unless underlying cause. Occasionally presents with complications, e.g. CVA, placental abruption.

E: General: ↑ BP (may be normal during first trimester resulting from normal decrease in early pregnancy). Retinopathy on fundal examination. Evidence of underlying cause if present, e.g. renal bruit, palpable kidneys, radiofemoral delay.

P: The blood flow to the uterus is increased in normal pregnancy owing to 40 % ↑ in cardiac output and 50 % ↓ systemic vascular resistance. This increase is not as great in hypertensive pregnancies compared to normotensive pregnancies because of the generalized vasospasm seen in essential hypertension, resulting in ↓ placental blood supply.

I: *Bloods*: FBC (haemoconcentration), U&E, serum urate, LFT (↑ transaminases), renal function. *Urine*: Dipstix (proteinuria), 24-h urinary metanephrines/vanillylmandelic acid (VMA) (exclude phaeochromocytoma). *Others*: Doppler of uterine arteries at 20–24 weeks (assess risk of pre-eclampsia), serial USS growth scans.

M: Pre-conception: assess risk (high risk if ≥ 1 of following present: > 40 years, > 15 year history of hypertension, BP = 160/110 mmHg, previous history of stillbirth, presence of diabetes, renal disease, CVS disease, connective tissue disease). *Advice*: lifestyle, medication (if on ACE inhibitors change to different drug).
During pregnancy: treat any underlying cause. Temporarily withdraw treatment if diastolic BP falls to < 110 mmHg. *Drugs*: methyldopa, nifedipine, labetalol. Avoid use of diuretics if possible. Monitor with fortnightly growth scans in third trimester. ↑ Observation for pre-eclampsia (proteinuria, ↑ urate levels).
Postnatal: ACE inhibitors are safe during puerperium.

C: Pre-eclampsia (20 %), placental abruption (1.5 %), IUGR, prematurity.

P: Maternal risks are mainly a result of development of pre-eclampsia. Perinatal risks are proportional to the level of hypertension, but therapeutic lowering of BP may compromise the fetus by ↓ placental perfusion.

Chronic pelvic pain syndrome

- **D:** Long-standing pelvic pain where no organic cause can be found.
- **A:** Unknown, associations as below.
- **A/R:** Depression; past history of pelvic disease; family history of pelvic disease; sexual dysfunction.
- **E:** Estimated 5–10 % gynaecology consultations.
- **H:** Long-standing pelvic pain (> 6 months duration); ? worse on standing/walking/with menstrual cycle; ? dysmenorrhoea; deep dyspareunia; emotional disturbance (? exacerbates pain).
- **E:** Often no abnormal finding on abdominal or pelvic examination. ? Cervix appears blue (due to congestion). Check for surgical causes/scars indicating previous surgery. ? Varicosities present.
- **P:** Congested pelvic veins found in some patients via pelvic venography/USS → ? indicates abnormal blood flow in response to certain stimuli → discomfort.
- **I:** Exclude pregnancy; MSU (? UTI); USS; laparoscopy.
- **M:** **If no pathology found**: reassurance; ? psychological intervention; ? antidepressants if appropriate; GnRH agonists; medroxyprogesterone acetate (↓ pelvic blood flow): ? NSAIDs or muscle relaxants; hysterectomy or bilateral ovarian vein ligation or embolization last resort. Randomized controlled trials suggest only antidepressants (fluoxetine) and GnRH agonists effective.
- **C:** Psychological sequelae.
- **P:** May resolve with little intervention or become a significant source of misery for some women.

Diabetes in pregnancy

D: Includes:
1 *Established diabetes* (DM): diabetes which existed prior to the pregnancy.
2 *Gestational diabetes* (GDM): glucose levels ↑ to diabetic levels during pregnancy and returning to normal following delivery.

A: DM: failure of the pancreas to produce insulin.
GDM: ↑ demand on pancreas revealing subclinical defects in carbohydrate metabolism.

A/R: DM: multifactorial.
GDM: family history, obesity, history of previous GDM, fetus >4kg or unexplained fetal death, ethnic groups (e.g. Asians), ↑ age, PCOS.

E: DM: 3–4 per 1000.
GDM: 2 per 100

H: DM: usually known to mother.
GDM: presents after second trimester. Often asymptomatic, symptoms include polydipsia, polyuria, recurrent UTI/*Candida*.

E: General: ↑ BP, oedema, retinopathy.
Abdomen: LGA (macrosomic fetus, polyhydramnios), malpresentation.

P: ↑ Insulin resistance occurs in pregnancy because of altered carbohydrate metabolism and ↑ secretion of HPL, progesterone and cortisol (insulin antagonists). Enhanced anabolism and catabolism can result in ↑ fluctuations of blood glucose (↑ risk of DKA and hypoglycaemia). Fluctuating glucose levels in the embryonic period may affect development → congenital abnormalities. Glucose crosses the placenta → fetal hyperinsulinaemia and macrosomia (insulin acts as a growth factor). Rebound hypoglycaemia is seen after birth as maternal glucose is withdrawn but the levels of insulin remain high.
 Fasting >7.8
I: GDM: *Diagnostic*: gold standard = 75g OGTT (positive if 2h level >7.8 mmol). *impaired glucose tolerance >11.2 → DM*.
Monitoring DM: Bloods: FBC, glucose, Hb A1c, U&E, RFT. Urine: microalbuminuria, MSU. Others: USS (fetal growth and congenital malformations), fundoscopy.

M: DM: *Preconceptual*: check renal function and retinopathy, optimize glucose control and give folic acid supplement.
DM/GDM: *During pregnancy*: (1) ↑ insulin as required (not usually needed in GDM). Avoid oral hypoglycaemics. (2) Detailed fetal anomaly scan at 18 weeks (DM only). (3) See in diabetic antenatal clinic every 2 weeks until 34 weeks, then weekly. Monitor fetal growth by USS. (4) Induce labour at 39 weeks (allow spontaneous labour in GDM if not severe). During labour give sliding scale insulin and 10% dextrose if required (established DM). CS if significant macrosomia. (5) Check newborn's glucose and U&E. Monitor closely. (6) Switch to prepregnancy insulin levels after delivery.

C: Diabetes: worsening of retinopathy, neuropathy and nephropathy, DKA, hypoglycaemia.
Pregnancy: ↑ risk of CS/instrumental delivery, hypertension, severe pre-eclampsia, polyhydramnios.
Fetus: congenital abnormalities (established DM only), e.g. sacral agenesis, cardiac/renal malformation, stillbirth, IUGR, prematurity, respiratory distress syndrome, macrosomia (shoulder dystocia). Neonate: hypoglycaemia, electrolyte disturbances, jaundice.

P: Rigid glucose control ↓ complications. 50% of those with GDM will develop diabetes within 10 years.

Dysfunctional uterine bleeding

- **D:** Heavy periods in the absence of identified pathology.
- **A:** **Anovulatory:** failure of follicular development and increased progesterone → cystic hyperplasia of the endometrium (unopposed oestrogen stimulation).
  Ovulatory: disturbed prostaglandin metabolism → increased prostaglandin E_2 (vasodilator) and decreased prostaglandin $F_{2\alpha}$ (vasoconstrictor).
- **A/R:** Extremes of reproductive age (anovulatory); ? association with obesity.
- **E:** Anovulatory 20 %; ovulatory 80 %.
- **H:** Debilitating menorrhagia; passage of clots; ? irregular periods; ? symptoms of PCOS.
- **E:** ? Signs of anaemia. Often no abnormalities on abdominal/pelvic examination.
- **P:** Anovulatory cycles: ? cystic glandular hyperplasia of the endometrium (thickened endometrium with cystic dilation of the endometrial glands and with hypertrophy of their columnar epithelium).
- **I:** Diagnosis of exclusion. *Bloods*: Hb (anaemia), (↓ platelets, rare cause),? clotting studies (e.g. family history clotting disorder, especially if soon after menarche); serum ferritin; TSH (only recommended if symptoms of thyroid disease). **USS** ? PCOS, fibroids, etc. **Hysteroscopy** and **endometrial biopsy** if necessary.
- **M:** Reassurance; advise on weight loss.
  Pharmacological: prostaglandin synthetase inhibitors (mefenamic acid); antifibrinolytics (tranexamic acid); COC pill; progestogens/progestogen-containing IUCD, e.g., Mirena.
  Surgical: endometrial ablation or hysterectomy if appropriate.
- **C:** Fe deficiency anaemia; social disturbance.
- **P:** Often controlled pharmacologically in younger women. However, surgical treatment may be preferred by older women who have completed their families.

Dysmenorrhoea

D: Lower abdominal pain felt just before or during menstruation. **Primary dysmenorrhoea (PD)**: no underlying pathology. **Secondary dysmenorrhoea (SD)**: identifiable underlying pathology.

A: PD: prostaglandin F2α (causes uterine hypercontractility and myometrial ischaemia).
SD: pelvic pathology/IUCD/pelvic congestion syndrome.

A/R: PD: family history, early menarche, heavy flow, psychological/social factors (affect severity).
SD: endometriosis, uterine retroversion, adenomyosis, PID, Asherman's syndrome, cervical stenosis, fibroids, endometrial polyp.

E: Most common gynaecological complaint. Affects 75% of women (20% severe).
PD: most common at 15–25 years of age.
SD: more common >30 years of age.

H: PD: onset usually within 24h before menstruation, resolves up to 48h later. Spasmodic lower abdominal/pelvic pain, radiates down anterior thigh (± lower back) ± nausea, vomiting, diarrhoea, fainting, fatigue, headache.
SD: Onset 2–3 days before menstruation, may be relieved when menstruation starts/late menstruation. ? Associated with menorrhagia/dyspareunia. Symptoms are specific to pathology (see pp. 3, 8, 33, 37, 59, 62).
Pelvic congestion syndrome—pain worse on standing and at night.

E: PD: no physical signs.
SD: depends on cause.
Pelvic congestion syndrome—vasocongestion (vagina/cervix), uterine enlargement + tenderness.

P: PD: no identifiable pathology.
SD: dependent on aetiology.

I: SD: pelvic USS, laparoscopy (uterine/adenexal mass/endometriosis).

M: PD: *First line*: NSAIDs (prostaglandin synthesis inhibition), e.g. mefenamic acid/ibuprofen/diclofenac sodium, OCP (ovulation suppression). *Second line*: progestogen (ovulation suppression), e.g. medroxyprogesterone acetate, GnRH analogue, e.g. goserelin, danazol (anti-oestrogenic, anti-progestogenic + androgen activity). Intractable dysmenorrhoea—psychiatric evaluation, surgery (hysterectomy—rare, only if family complete).
SD: treat underlying cause, NSAIDs.

C: Limitation of daily activity, school/work absenteeism.

P: PD: 95% of women gain relief with NSAIDs/OCP. May also improve spontaneously/with childbirth.

Dyspareunia

D: Recurrent pelvic pain felt during or after sexual intercourse.

A: Organic or psychological aetiology.

A/R: **Organic:** *Superficial*: infection (vulva, vagina, Bartholin's gland), dermatological disorder (vulva, vagina), congenitally narrow hymenal ring, vaginal stenosis, vaginal septum, painful scarring, postmenopausal atrophy (vagina), inadequate lubrication, vaginismus, vulval vestibulitis syndrome.
Deep: pelvic infections, endometriosis, pelvic masses, fixed uterine retroversion, postoperative scarring, bladder/bowel pathology, chronic constipation.
Psychological: intrapersonal conflict (previous traumatic experience, e.g. sexual abuse, guilt about sexuality, lack of sexual knowledge, fear of sexually transmitted disease/pregnancy, emotional disorder), interpersonal conflict (relationship problem), failure of arousal response.

E: 30–50 % of gynaecological patients experiencing sexual problems.

H: Superficial/deep pain during or after sexual intercourse ± other symptoms specific to organic cause, pelvic pain, failure of arousal response, relationship difficulty, psychosexual problems.

E: General, abdominal, vulvovaginal and pelvic examination may be helpful for signs of infection, narrow hymen, vaginal stenosis, vaginal septum, episotomy scarring, atrophic vaginitis. Also look for signs of above mentioned deep pathologies, e.g., pelvic mass. Occasionally, there are no signs (psychological cause).

P: Varies according to cause.

I: FBC, HVS, endocervical swab or *Chlamydia* swabs may be indicated. Pelvic USS and diagnostic laparoscopy may be required.

M: **Organic:** topical steroids (dermatological condition), local anaesthetic gel, HRT/topical oestrogen/vaginal lubricant (vaginal dryness), antibiotics/antifungal (infection), low dose amitriptyline, adapt sexual position, surgery (hymen/vaginal/scar abnormality), treat underlying pathology.
Psychological: reassurance, psychological/sexual counselling, psychotherapy, psychiatric evaluation (complex psychosexual problems), hymenal-vaginal dilation (vaginismus).

C: Relationship difficulties, psychological disturbance, complications specific to organic cause.

P: **Organic:** good prognosis following treatment.
Psychological: worse prognosis as difficult to treat.

Ectopic pregnancy

D: Pregnancy outside the uterine cavity.

A: Delay in passage of conceptus along fallopian tube.

A/R: Previous tubal surgery (restoration of tubal patency, sterilization); previous ectopic pregnancy, fertility treatment (GIFT, IVF); peritubal adhesions (endometriosis, PID, appendicitis); congenital abnormalities (e.g. diverticula), IUCD, progesterone only pill, emergency contraceptive pill, luteal phase defects, ↑ age.

E: ↑ Incidence, currently is approx 1 in 150 pregnancies in white population, 1 in 100 pregnancies in non-white population.

H: 20 % present acutely, 80 % subacutely.
Acute: acute, severe, lower abdominal pain, possibly referred to shoulder tip, syncope.
Subacute: (less defined symptoms make diagnosis more difficult): amenorrhoea (4–10 weeks) lower abdominal pain, PV bleeding—scanty, dark 'prune juice'.

E: *Acute:* shock: pale, cold, clammy, tachycardic, hypotensive. Lower abdominal peritonism (distension, guarding and rebound tenderness). *Bimanual*: adnexal tenderness/mass (may be hidden by guarding), uterus enlarged but smaller than expected for dates, cervical excitation, external os closed.
Subacute: peritoneal irritation. *Bimanual*: as for acute, but signs less defined.

P: Mechanical obstruction or cilia dysfunction may result in implantation of the blastocyst in the fallopian tube (95 %—ampulla most common site). Less common: ovary, uterus (cornu, cervix, rudimentary horn), broad ligament, abdominal cavity. Pregnancy ends by tubal abortion (65 %) (conceptus is expelled into tube), tubal rupture (35 %) or by secondary abdominal/broad ligament pregnancy (rare).

I: *Acute: Bloods*: FBC (↓ Hb), ESR, CRP (infection), clotting, group and save, U&E, amylase (↑). *Urine*: β-hCG. *Others*: consider USS, but may not have time to arrange for one.
Subacute: Bloods: FBC (↓ Hb). *Urine*: β-hCG. *Others*: USS—will either confirm intrauterine pregnancy, tubal pregnancy (features may include: tubal rupture, live tubal pregnancy, tubal abortion, intrauterine pseudogestational sac) or no diagnosis reached. For latter group: serum rapid sensitive β-hCG. If levels > 1000 IU/L, intrauterine pregnancy should be seen on TV USS. If levels < 1000 IU/L and patient haemodynamically stable, repeat in 48 h. If risen by > 66 % early (< 5 weeks) intrauterine pregnancy is likely.

M: *Acute:* resuscitate. Transfer to theatre immediately for laparotomy and salpingectomy.
Subacute: Medical: 80–90 % success rate. Consider if diagnosed unruptured, non-viable, ectopic pregnancy < 4 cm and serum hCG < 1500 IU/L. Methotrexate either systemically or direct injection into fallopian tube under USS guidance. Follow-up: β-hCG and TV USS every 1–2 days to ensure termination. *Surgical*: laparoscopy and salpingectomy or salpingostomy. Anti-D given to all Rhesus-negative women.

C: Rupture resulting in massive haemorrhage, infertility, complications of pelvic surgery, psychological effects.

P: Other tube normal: 80 % chance intrauterine pregnancy; 10 % chance further ectopic.
Other tube diseased: 50 % chance intrauterine pregnancy; > 10 % chance further ectopic.

Endometriosis

D: Presence of normal functioning endometrial tissue outside the uterus.

A: Unknown. Current theories include the following:
1 *Sampson*: retrograde menstruation results in implantation of endometrial cells in the peritoneal cavity, which then undergo the normal cycle of proliferation and bleeding each month. This is only a prerequisite, as retrograde menstruation occurs in all women. Survival and proliferation of tissue may be caused by an underlying defect in cell-mediated immunity.
2 *Meyer*: metaplastic induction factor induces metaplasia of coelomic epithelium.
3 *Szlacter*: presence of endometriosis in scar tissue is a result of unintentional transfer of endometrial tissue during surgery.
4 *Halban*: endometriosis occurring at distant sites is brought about by endometrial cell spread via lymph and blood vessels.

A/R: White population, fourth decade, delayed child bearing. Rare in Afro-Caribbeans.

E: Up to 25 % of women.

H: Asymptomatic. *Pelvic involvement*: cyclical, lower abdominal, colicky pain occurring premenstrually and reaching peak at onset of menstruation. Dyspareunia. Subfertility. Menstrual disorders uncommon except with ovary involvement. May present acutely with rupture of endometrioma. *Bowel involvement*: colicky abdominal pain, PR bleeding. *Bladder involvement*: haematuria. *Distant sites (rare)*: haemoptysis, epistaxis.

E: Usually unremarkable.
Pelvic: Bimanual: thick nodules of varying size. Fixed and retroverted uterus (severe disease).

P: Macro: lesions seen as white, red, black or brown according to level of activity. Common sites include: uterosacral ligaments, ovary and pelvic peritoneum. Less common sites include: fallopian tubes, bowel, lower genital tract, urinary tract, scar tissue and distant sites, e.g. lungs, nose.
Micro: ectopic endometrium surrounded by stroma form cysts and respond to the cyclical levels of progesterone and oestrogen. During menstruation the ectopic endometrium bleeds into itself, and blood becomes trapped. The cycle recurs each month so that as more blood is shed the cyst grows and is filled with tarry, chocolate-coloured blood ('chocolate' cyst). Cysts may be attacked by haemosiderin-laden macrophages. Larger cysts may infiltrate adjacent structures causing fibrosis and adhesions.

I: *Bloods*: FBC (↓ Hb), ESR, CRP (PID), Ca 125 (↑ as a result of peritoneal irritation). *Others*: pelvic USS (ovarian cysts—endometriomas), laparoscopy (diagnostic).

M: No treatment if symptomless. If symptomatic consider:
Medical: (1) NSAIDs for pain; (2) OCP; (3) LHRH analogues, e.g. *goserelin* in conjunction with continuous oestrogen (↓ hypo-oestrogenic side-effects); (4) anti-progesterone (e.g. *gestrinone*); (5) *danazol* (synthetic steroid, but poorly tolerated because of side-effects such as virilization).
Surgery (if above fails): electrodiathermy or laser vaporization of lesions. Cystectomy or drainage and lasering of base for cysts. Consider hysterectomy as a last resort.

C: Rupture of cyst, subfertility, sexual dysfunction.

P: Improvement of symptoms seen in up to 80 %, but recurrence within 2 years occurs in 20 %. Symptoms usually subside at the menopause.

Endometritis

D: Inflammation of the endometrium resulting from acute or chronic infection.

A: Childbirth and instrumentation; ascending sexually acquired infection (from the cervix); haematogenous spread of infection (e.g. tuberculosis); spread of infection from other pelvic organs (in PID); termination of pregnancy.

A/R: Premature rupture of membranes, instrumental delivery, CS, abortion (especially backstreet), excessive curettage, foreign body, retained products of conception, advanced cervical/endometrial carcinoma, postmenopausal atrophy (atrophic endometritis—loss of vaginal acidity and ↑ ascending infection). Associated infection of other pelvic organs would change diagnosis to PID.

E: Dependent on aetiology and the patient population.

H: May be asymptomatic, vaginal discharge, irregular menstruation, dyspareunia (see also PID, p. 57).
Chronic infection: secondary infertility, secondary amenorrhea, low-grade pelvic pain.
Puerperal infection: abdominal discomfort, malaise, fever, offensive lochia.

E: Uterine tenderness (on internal examination) (see also PID, p. 57).

P: Infection and inflammation of the endometrium. Uterine adhesions (chronic infection).
Pathogens: *Chlamydia trachomatis, Neisseria gonorrhoea, Mycobacterium tuberculosis*, actinomycosis (from IUCD) staphylococcus, streptococcus.

I: *Bloods*: FBC, ESR, CRP.
Endometrial biopsy/dilation and curettage (end menstrual cycle).
Endocervical swab (chlamydia ELISA, bacterial culture and antibiotic sensitivity).

M: 14–21-day course of broad-spectrum antibiotic (effectiveness not proven).

C: PID, Asherman's syndrome, infertility, miscarriage, pyometra.

P: Most cases resolve with adequate antibiotic therapy.

Epilepsy in pregnancy

D: A seizure is the paroxysmal discharge of cerebral neurones resulting in convulsions. Epilepsy is the continuing tendency to have seizures. Epilepsy can be affected by pregnancy and visa versa.

A: Effects on epilepsy: pre-existing epilepsy can be made worse by altered pharmacokinetics of anticonvulsants (dilution, ↓ absorption, ↑ metabolism of anticonvulsants) and compliance issues (fear of congenital abnormalities caused by drugs).
Effects on pregnancy: congenital abnormalities can be a result of genetic factors, hypoxia during grand mal fits and anticonvulsant drugs (partly because of interference with folic acid levels).

A/R: Effects on epilepsy: ↑ seizure frequency and severity is more likely with secondary generalized or complex partial epilepsy.
Effects on pregnancy: ↑ incidence of congenital abnormality is more likely with multidrug regimens, phenytoin and sodium valproate.

E: Co-exists in ∼1% of pregnancies. One-third will have ↑ seizures, one-third will remain the same, and one-third will have an improvement in condition.

H: Recurrent seizures, non-compliance.

E: Usually unremarkable.

P: n/a

I: *Bloods*: FBC, MCV, serum and red cell folate (exclude folate deficiency). Serum anticonvulsant levels, LFT. *Others*: detailed fetal anomaly scan at 18–22 weeks (neural tube, cardiac and orofacial abnormalities).

M: Pre-pregnancy: aim for single drug regimen or, if seizure free for 2–3 years, consider withdrawal. Consider changing to less teratogenic drug (e.g. carbamazepine). Emphasize risk to fetus of non-compliance. 5 mg/day oral folate supplement.
Pregnancy: continue folate supplements to at least 12 weeks. 20 mg vitamin K PO from 36 weeks for women on carbamazepine, phenytoin, primidone or phenobarbital (enzyme-inducing drugs). Manage seizures accordingly (most are self-limiting, but if prolonged give diazepam PR). If this fails consider IV phenytoin and, in extreme cases, ventilation).
Postnatal: give neonate 1 g vitamin K IM after delivery. *Advice*: breastfeeding is safe. Educate about protective bathing and feeding. Warn that anticonvulsants ↓ effectiveness of OCP so higher dose is needed.

C: Epilepsy: status epilepticus. *Pregnancy*: ↑ incidence of placental abruption (3 ×), vaginal bleeding, interventional delivery, breech presentation, congenital abnormalities (especially CVS (4 ×), orofacial (6 ×) and neural tube defects (most common with sodium valproate (1.5%)). Severe cases of pre-eclampsia are more common in epileptics. ↑ Risk of haemorrhagic disease of newborn (anticonvulsants ↓ vitamin K levels).

P: Preconceptual care and specialist management during pregnancy minimizes incidence of complications.

Fetal distress in labour

D: An indication of fetal hypoxia, with or without acidosis. Diagnosis is by intermittent auscultation with a Pinnard, continuous CTG or by meconium staining of liquor.

A: With each uterine contraction venous blood flow is obstructed prior to arterial. Intervillous blood flow is impaired. Prolonged contractions and placental insufficiency reduce fetal reserve and result in hypoxia, hypercapnia and respiratory acidosis (compounded by metabolic acidosis). Sympathetic activity →↑ FHR. Persistent hypoxia → bradycardia (vagally mediated).

A/R: Failure of labour to progress; meconium aspiration (also complication); hypertonic uterus; placental insufficiency; intrauterine infection; cord prolapse; placental abruption; IUGR and prior fetal compromise (e.g. following recurrent APH, pre-eclampsia, hypertensive disorders, diabetes).

E: 2–10 % incidence. More common with IUGR (↓ glycogen stores).

H: History and/or symptoms relating to underlying condition(s).

E: Signs of maternal exhaustion with prolonged labour; fundal palpation → ? ↑ strength and frequency of uterine contractions; assess for cephalopelvic disproportion, cervical dilation, state of membranes, presentation, station and position of presenting part, cord prolapse; ? meconium staining of liquor (graded from I to III), ? oligohydramnios (? PROM, prior fetal compromise).

P: n/a

I: Continuous CTG (NB debate over benefits in low risk): baseline tachycardia (> 160 bpm)/bradycardia(< 100 bpm), ↓ variability, late decelerations; in association with fetal scalp sampling: assess hypoxia and acidaemia—falling pH < 7.2 first stage, < 7.15 second stage. Maternal FBC and group and save serum (if CS envisaged).

M: Significant hypoxia necessitates delivery (? CS/instrumental).

C: Fetal: death/brain damage below pH 6.9; ischaemic damage to organs; ↑ seizures; passage of meconium (? vagally mediated loss of anal sphincter tone) ? → meconium aspiration into the lungs (NB fetal distress → reflex gasping).
Maternal: complications of an operative delivery, e.g. haemorrhage, haematoma, infection.

P: Dependent on the underlying cause and adequacy of intervention.

Fibroids (leiomyomas)

D: Benign tumours of uterine myometrium.

A: Unknown. ? Action of oestrogen and progesterone on uterine smooth muscle. ? DNA damage (many fibroids have chromosomal abnormalities).

A/R: Nulliparity, obesity, black women. ↑ Growth in pregnancy.↓ Risk with smoking, OCP and multiparity.

E: Up to one-third women > 30 years.

H: Asymptomatic (50 %). Menorrhagia (one-third, especially submucosal fibroids), IMB (especially intramural), anaemia, pressure effects (urinary frequency, tenesmus, oedema of leg (as a result of pressure on common iliac vein), pain, infertility. May present acutely with pelvic pain (caused by torsion or red degeneration).

E: Abdomen: distension.
Pelvic: *Bimanual*: asymmetrical/nodular uterine enlargement. Non-tender uterus except if undergoing red degeneration (more common in pregnancy). Cervical displacement.

P: Macro: can be intramural, subserosal or submucosal.
Micro: consist of whorled, smooth muscle layers interspersed with connective tissue. Can undergo secondary changes including the following.
1 *Hyaline degeneration*: deposition of mucopolysaccharide around the muscle fibres. Most common change.
2 *Calcification*: common after menopause.
3 *Red degeneration*: bland coagulative necrosis. Most common in pregnancy.
4 *Cystic change*: liquefaction and cystic areas.

I: Bloods: FBC (↑ / ↓). *Others*: pelvic USS, hysteroscopy and laparoscopy (if large).

M: Treat only symptomatic cases.
Medical: normal treatment for menorrhagia (e.g. NSAIDs/OCP) may not be successful for control of symptoms caused by fibroids. Consider: *GnRH analogue* (use for max 6 months because of risk of osteoporosis). Can ↓ size and vascularity of fibroid, so suitable prior to surgery. Fibroid may grow after withdrawal of treatment.
Surgical: options include: (1) removal at hysteroscopy if small; (2) myomectomy (↑ risk of haemorrhage); (3) uterine artery embolization; (4) hysterectomy (as last resort).

C: Iron-deficiency anaemia, polycythaemia (giant leiomyomas), torsion and infarction, subfertility, malignant change → leiomyosarcoma (0.5 %).
Pregnancy: red degeneration, fetal obstruction, malpresentation, PPH, puerperal infection.

P: Tend to be larger and more problematic with ↑ age and pregnancy. Usually shrink and undergo calcification after the menopause (↓ oestrogen). Recurrence after treatment (except hysterectomy) is ~1 %.

Genital warts (condylomata acuminata)

D: Benign growths of the vulva, cervix or vagina caused by infection with human papilloma virus.

A: Sexually transmited human papilloma virus infection (primarily subtypes 6 and 11, occasionally types 16 and 18).

A/R: Multiple sexual partners, partner with previous multiple sexual partners.
Florid lesions: diabetes mellitus, pregnancy, OCP, immunosuppression.

E: 5–10 % sexually active adults infected annually (estimated). 10 % infected women develop clinical evidence of disease.

H: Asymptomatic (most cases). Vulval lesions (painless, slow growing), pruritus, burning, tenderness (site of lesion), vaginal discharge, superficial dyspareunia (vaginal warts).

E: Frequently multiple raised papillomatous/flat lesions of the vulva, vagina and cervix/clinically undetectable.

P: Papillomatous, flat, spiked or inverted lesions.
Papillomatous lesions: raised lesion, finger-like projections, often contain capillaries.
Flat lesions: clinically undetectable, granular surface, mosaic pattern (on colposcopy).
Spiked lesions: hyperkeratotic lesions, with surface projections and capillary tips.
Inverted lesions: (rare) found on cervix, grow into cervical glands.

I: Biopsy (atypical lesion), cervical smear + cytology (if last smear >3 years before), colposcopy + biopsy (cervical lesions).

M: Outpatient application of podophyllin 1–2 times per week or podophyllotoxin solution b.d. in 3-day cycle, for 4 weeks.
Resistant/extensive lesions: cryotherapy/laser therapy/electocautery/scissor excision. Consider interferon/topical immune stimulant (imiquimod) if immunosuppressed.
Advise barrier contraception (during treatment + further 3 months + with new sexual partners). Trace and examine recent sexual contacts.
Pregnant women: cannot use podophyllin, use alternative treatment, consider CS if large vaginal/introitus lesions present.

C: Infection of confluent lesions, recurrence, CIN, cervical carcinoma, vulval carcinoma (rare), laryngeal papillomatosis (in neonate of infected mother).

P: Recurrence common for weeks to months (50–60 % with podophyllin treatment). 1.5 % risk of cervical carcinoma.

Gestational trophoblastic malignancy

D: Includes invasive mole and choriocarcinoma.

A: Abnormal chromosomal material of placental tissue. Invasive mole is always preceded by hydatidiform mole. Choriocarcinoma may be preceded by hydatidiform mole (50 %), normal pregnancy (25 %), other pregnancy, e.g. abortion, ectopic (25 %).

A/R: See hydatidiform mole (p. 41).
Invasive mole: complete mole > partial mole.
Choriocarcinoma: complete mole, ↑ age.

E: Rare. Invasive mole more common than choriocarcinoma. 1 % partial moles → invasive moles. 10 % complete moles → invasive, 3 % → choriocarcinoma.
1 in 10 000 normal pregnancies → choriocarcinoma.

H: Following molar pregnancy and ERPC: persistent vaginal bleeding, often heavy. Nausea. Lower abdominal pain (severe and sudden onset if uterine rupture (rare). Metastatic symptoms (especially lungs), e.g. pleuritic pain, haemoptysis. Symptoms of thyrotoxicosis (rare).
Following non-molar pregnancy: occasionally presents months or years following pregnancy with symptoms as above. In addition—amenorrhoea and subfertility.

E: Acute: shock, lower abdominal peritonism (if intra-abdominal haemorrhage resulting from uterine rupture).
Chronic: *Abdomen*: distension, uterine enlargement. *Pelvic inspection*: vagina–swelling, metastasis (dense red areas, bleed easily and occur mainly at introitus). Uterine bleeding. *Bimanual*: uterus—enlarged, tender.

P: Invasive mole: as for hydatidiform mole but with myometrial invasion (diagnostic feature).
Choriocarcinoma: epithelial tumour of syncytio-and cytotrophoblastic cells (arranged in sheets or foci). Poorly differentiated, absent villi and invasion of muscles and blood vessels.

I: Serum β-hCG: following ERPC for molar pregnancy suspect malignancy if persistently raised or rising levels of serum β-hCG 6–8 weeks after procedure. Following non-molar pregnancy levels may be grossly ↑ (> 100 000 IU/L). Exclude if levels < 2 IU/L.
Others: *Bloods*: FBC (↓ Hb), clotting, U&E, LFT (metastasis), TFT (thyrotoxicosis). *Diagnostic*: pelvic USS (snowstorm appearance of uterus/multiple cystic or vesicular appearance, exclude pregnancy). *Exclude metastasis*: CXR, CT chest and abdomen.

M: In specialist centre (three in UK: Charing Cross in London, Sheffield and Edinburgh). Chemotherapy main treatment as tumour very chemosensitive. Categorize patients according to risk. *High risk*: combination chemotherapy—methotrexate and actinomycin or etoposide. *Low risk*: methotrexate.
Follow-up: monitor β-hCG levels to ensure ↓. Follow-up at regular intervals for life (risk of recurrence of choriocarcinoma).
Advice: avoid pregnancy and COC pill for 1 year.

C: Metastasis: more common with choriocarcinoma. Lungs most common. Less commonly to GI tract and liver. Uterine perforation, recurrence of choriocarcinoma.

P: Very good. 100 % cure for low-risk patients, 80 % cure for high-risk patients. Majority go on to have subsequent successful pregnancy.

Gonorrhoea infection in female genital tract

D: Sexually transmitted infection caused by *Neisseria gonorrhoeae*.

A: Sexual intercourse with infected partner (75 % transmission rate).

A/R: Unprotected intercourse, multiple partners, intercourse with high-risk partner, young age (< 25 years), urban women, presence of other STIs.

E: Increasing since 1994. 17 000 cases in 1999 in UK.

H: Incubation period 2–10 days. Two-thirds asymptomatic.
Classic early symptoms:
1 *urethritis*: severe dysuria (pain on urination—worse at start), frequency;
2 *cervicitis*: purulent, offensive vaginal discharge.
Complications: *Local spread*: bartholinitis (see p. 11), skenitis (infection of Skene's glands). *Ascending spread*: salpingitis—fever, malaise, lower abdominal pain. *Disseminated:* (septicaemia and arthritis) fever, malaise, rash, tenosynovitis.
Rare: infection of rectum or pharynx (usually asymptomatic) or perihepatitis (Fitz-Hugh–Curtis syndrome) which presents with right upper abdominal pain that is worse on coughing.

E: **General** (if ascending spread or dissemination): pyrexia > 39°C, tachycardia, dehydration, joint tenderness and swelling, distal purple macular rash. Suspect disseminated gonococcal infection in any young person presenting with tenosynovitis and fever.
Abdomen: lower abdominal tenderness and peritonism.
Pelvic: white/yellow purulent discharge, abscess (urethral or Bartholin's). *Speculum*: acute cervicitis with mucopurulent discharge. *Bimanual*: uterine tenderness, adnexal tenderness, cervical excitation.

P: Intracellular aerobic Gram-negative kidney-shaped diplococci seen in pairs (facing each other). Infects the columnar and transitional epithelium of genitourinary tract (it is unable to penetrate the stratified squamous epithelium of the vagina). Highly fastidious organism. Diagnosis is based on a Gram stain of appropriate swab (50 % sensitivity) followed by culture on special nutrient medium (e.g. Thayer-Martin) and chocolate agar.

I: *Bloods*: FBC (↑ WCC), ESR, blood culture. Screen for other sexually transmitted diseases (syphilis, HIV, hepatitis). *Urine*: β-hCG (exclude pregnancy), MSU (exclude infection).
STI screen: vaginal swab (*Trichomonas vaginalis*, bacterial vaginosis, *Candida*), endocervical swab (gonorrhoea, *Chlamydia*) and urethral, rectal and pharyngeal swabs (gonorrhoea). Microscopy and culture of swab will identify *N. gonorrhoea* and antibiotic sensitivity (usually sensitive to penicillin).

M: **Advice:** contact partner(s) for contact tracing.
Treatment: admit if disseminated disease. If uncomplicated: penicillin and probenecid. If resistant to penicillin: ampicillin, cephalosporin or spectomycin. Continue treatment for several days until symptoms have resolved if upper genital tract involvement. Re-screen after 7 days.

C: **Ascending infection:** PID (15 %) and subfertility.
Disseminated infection: septicaemia, arthritis, meningitis, endocarditis, Fitz-Hugh–Curtis syndrome (rare). Adult ophthalmitis (rare).
Pregnancy: miscarriage, IUGR, prematurity, IUD, post-partum sepsis.
Neonate: neonatal ophthalmia (presents 2–7 days after birth with severe bilateral conjunctivitis).

P: Good if correct treatment.

Hydatidiform mole

D: Benign tumour of trophoblastic tissue.

A: Abnormal fertilization (enucleated ovum and/or duplicated haploid sperm, or dispermy).
Partial mole: triploid conceptus (maternal component retained).
Complete mole: diploid containing only paternal genes (duplicated haploid sperm/dispermy).

A/R: Extremes of reproductive age; Philippino/Japanese/oriental origin, previous history.

E: Rare, 1 in 2000 pregnancies in the UK.

H: Towards end first trimester: vaginal bleeding ± excessive vomiting, uterine contractions, expulsion of grape-like vesicles/asymptomatic. Rarely: signs of hyperemesis, pre eclampsia, thyrotoxicosis.

E: Soft, boggy uterus larger than expected for gestational age. Absent fetal heart sounds (ultrasonic fetal heart monitor). ? Enlarged ovaries (theca/lutein cysts). ? Signs of pre-eclampsia.

P: Macro: 'bunch of grapes' appearance. Confined to uterus. Complete moles replace the placenta, no fetus found. Partial moles partially replaces the placenta, fetus may be present (early first trimester).
Micro: trophoblastic hyperplasia, hydropic villi, vesicle formation, decreased or absent blood vessels within the villi.

I: Blood: serum β-hCG (greatly elevated), TFT, 4 units cross-matched blood.
Urine: β-hCG (greatly elevated). USS: fetal absence, characteristic vesicular pattern (snowstorm appearance).

M: Replace blood loss. Empty uterus by suction evacuation intact mole/aspiration and curettage (evidence of spontaneous evacuation). Syntometrine (minimize bleeding). Hysterectomy (fertility not desired/intraperitoneal haemorrhage). Histological analysis of specimen. Notification of regional centres (Charing Cross, Sheffield, Dundee) for inclusion in Trophoblastic Disease Register. Regular follow-up (urine β-hCG—2 weekly until normal, then less often for 6 months–1 year) for 1 year (co-ordinated by regional centres). Pregnancy contraindicated during this time (β-hCG may mask malignancy).

C: Malignant change to non-metastatic invasive mole or metastatic choriocarcinoma.

P: Good—malignant change rare (5 % complete moles).

Hyperemesis gravidarum

D: Persistent nausea and vomiting in the first trimester necessitating hospital admission.

A: Unknown. Excessively high hCG levels suggested resulting from associations with molar and multiple pregnancy. ? Reflects better implantation → higher hormone levels (? therefore associated with improved outcome). Adrenal disease also suggested. Associated with thyroid disease—↑ hCG can → hyperthyroidism but no evidence that thyroid disease per se causes hyperemesis.

A/R: Youth; primigravidae; previous history; multiple pregnancy; molar pregnancy; thyroid/adrenal dysfunction; social/psychological factors.

E: Rare, 1 in 1000.

H: Severe nausea and vomiting; anorexia; dehydration; weight loss; symptoms relating to complications.

E: General: dehydration, signs of jaundice or anaemia.
Abdominal palpation: ↑ fundal height (? multiple pregnancy); tenderness indicating another cause; auscultate for bowel sounds (surgical cause), fetal heart (multiple/molar pregnancy).

P: n/a   Blood urea & haematocrit ↑↑—dehydration

I: Bloods: FBC: Hb—anaemia (resulting from anorexia); WCC—exclude infection; PCV—dehydration; U&E electrolyte imbalance, renal function; LFT especially if jaundiced; TFT; β-hCG ↑ ++ in molar pregnancy. Urine: urinalysis—exclude UTI, for ketonuria. Other: USS—for twin/molar pregnancy.

M: Admit: antiemetics (e.g. prochlorperazine PR; metaclopramide 10 mg/8 h IV); IV hydration with saline; vitamin supplements including thiamine (prevent Wernicke's encephalopathy); psychological support.
Severe cases: Iso-osmolar feeds; regular gastric aspiration; ? TPN.
Monitor: fluid balance; blood glucose if ketones evident on UA.
Advise: on diet—small frequent snacks, avoid spicy, fatty foods.
Follow-up: monitor maternal weight gain and fetal growth.

C: Severe vomiting may → hypovolaemia, electrolyte disturbance, polyneuritis (deficit of B vitamins), liver failure, renal failure.

P: Most settle with minimal care. Uncontrolled cases may respond to corticosteroids.

Infertility

D: Inability to conceive after 1 year of unprotected intercourse. **Primary**—no previous pregnancies; **secondary**—previously successful pregnancy(ies).

A: Multiple.
Female:
1 *Idiopathic*.
2 *Tubal disease*: → blockage/damage cilia.
3 *Anovulation*: PCOS most common cause; also menopause/perimenopause, premature menopause; more rarely, pituitary disease (e.g. *previous sickness* adenoma → hyperprolactinaemia → disruption pulsatile gonadotrophin release), thyroid disorders (alter ovulatory cycle → menstrual dysfunction), adrenal dysfunction; rarely, lack of follicular FSH receptors, ovary unresponsive to gonadotrophins.
4 *Endometriosis*: mechanical distortion of tubes, ovarian destruction. *- chocolate cyst*
5 *Other*: fibroids (physical hindrance); Asherman's syndrome; antisperm antibodies in cervical mucus (→ agglutination/immoblization); resistant ovary syndrome (rare), anorexia nervosa, psychological factors (alter hypothalamic function).
Male: varicocele, undescended testes, heat/trauma, retrograde ejaculation, oligo/azospermia, antisperm antibodies, mumps, epididymal/vas obstruction, chromosomal abnormalities. *absent vas def → CystcFib*

A/R: Age >35 years; excessive weight loss (HPO dysfunction—hypogonadotrophic hypogonadism); obesity; oligo/amenorrhoea.

E: Affects 10–15 % couples of which: 25 % idiopathic, 25 % male causes, 25 % anovulatory, 20 % tubal problems, 5 % other.

H: Inability to conceive. ? Amenorrhoea/oligomenorrhoea. ? Symptoms of underlying disorders, e.g. PCOS. ? Decreased coital frequency. ? History of pelvic/genital surgery/infection. ? Irradiation.

E: **Male:** testes (presence, size, signs of infection—also prostate).
Female: pelvic (exclude pelvic pathology, malformations, pregnancy).

P: As for specific aetiologies.

I: **Male:** 2 × seminal fluid analysis 6 weeks apart (sperm density, morphology, motility, antisperm antibodies); FSH; ? karyotype; testicular biopsy.
Female: *Ovulation*: 21 day progesterone (daily temperature recording/spinnbarkeit unreliable), LH:FSH ratio (PCOS). *Tubal patency*: chromotubation—hysterosalpingogram (radio-opaque dye injected through cervix should spill into peritoneal cavity), hysterosalpingo-contrast ultrasound (echocontrast medium injected through cervix detected via ultrasound); ? laparoscopy. *Sperm penetration of cervical mucus*: post-coital test (midcycle, examine sperm in sample of endocervical cervical mucus 6–12 h after coitus)—increasingly discredited.

M: **Medical:** clomifene (anti-oestrogen—stimulates follicular maturation) 50 mg/day (increase to 150 mg/day) from day 2–6 cycle, intercourse midcycle; ? administer hCG when follicle 16–18 mm diameter with ultrasound monitoring; gonadotrophins—FSH/LH IM (hypothalamopituitary dysfunction) ? with hCG; IV/SC pulsatile GnRH (hypogonadotrophic hypogonadism); dopamine agonists, e.g. bromocriptine (hyperprolactinaemia).
Surgical: *Tubal disease*: salpingolysis (remove adhesions), reversal of sterilization, cornual re-anastomosis (dissecting blocked segment and joining the cut ends), salpingotomy (? laser, opening and fixing of fimbrial end).
Other: fibroid removal.

Infertility continued

Other: intrauterine insemination (IUI) semen injected through cervix via cannula, ? concomitant gonadotrophins; IVF—sperm (masturbation) and egg (ovarian stimulation and egg collection) brought into contact *in vitro* → embryo transfer; ICSI—? more efficient; GIFT—collected eggs and semen → fallopian tube; ? weight correction; psychotherapy.

C: Psychological sequelae; ovarian hyperstimulation with induction of ovulation; side-effects of treatments, ovarian cancer (? caused by fertility treatments; or may be related to infertility/low parity).

P: Dependent on underlying aetiology, significant source of distress for many couples, treatment may be protracted.

Repeated ux of preg fail → pre-implantation genetic diagnosis

Intrauterine death

D: Death of fetus *in utero* after 24 weeks' gestation.

A: *Fetal:* congenital abnormalities (e.g. neural tube defects, hydrops, congenital heart disease), chromosomal abnormalities, infection (especially parvo B19 and *Listeria*).
Others: Vascular: antepartum haemorrhage, twin–twin transfusion syndrome, placental insufficiency. *Infection:* maternal (especially parvo B19 and *Listeria*), placental (chorioamniitis). *Trauma:* uterine rupture. *Autoimmune:* SLE, antiphospholipid antibodies. *Metabolic:* diabetes. *Intrapartum complications:* dystocia, obstructed labour, birth asphyxia. *Idiopathic. Cord:* compression, strangulation, prolapse.

A/R: Previous history, multiple pregnancy (especially monochorionic), hypertension, smoking, excess alcohol, extremes of maternal age, post-term, ↑ AFP and β-hCG during early pregnancy, ↑ or ↓ liquor, fetal growth restriction or small for dates.

E: 5 in 1000 deliveries.

H: ↓ Or absent fetal movements, pregnancy feels 'different' (patient may no longer 'feel' pregnant). May present acutely, e.g. antepartum haemorrhage.

E: **Abdomen:** ↓ symphysio-fundal height. Unable to detect fetal heart with Pinnards or hand-held Doppler.

P: Depends on cause. Autopsy alone determines cause in 1 in 5 cases.

I: **Before delivery:** USS to confirm fetal death. *Bloods:* FBC (Hb, WCC), ESR, CRP (infection), Hb A1c, blood glucose (diabetes), clotting (DIC); LFT; lupus anticoagulant and anticardiolipin antibodies (autoimmune disease); Kleihauer test (feto-maternal transfusion); infections screen (parvo B19, *Listeria*; toxoplasmosis, rubella, CMV, hepatitis (TORCH)).
After delivery: detailed examination of baby, placenta, cord and membranes. Blood sample from cord for karyotyping and infection screen. Autopsy if parental consent.

M: **Labour:** 80% labour spontaneously within 2 weeks, but IOL is usually performed for psychological reasons. *Medical:* intravaginal prostaglandins or misoprostol given. Epidural is standard unless abnormal clotting. When >4 cm dilated and established labour, perform amniotomy. *Psychological:* ensure support. Encourage presence of partner. When baby is born, encourage parents to see, touch and spend time alone with their baby, and take photographs.
Post delivery: *Medical:* bromocriptine to suppress lactation. *Psychological:* arrange for specialist counselling and give details of local support groups. Some hospitals have an annual memorial service for parents who have lost a baby. Discuss consent for autopsy. Arrange follow-up with consultant in 4–6 weeks to discuss results of autopsy, if consented, or any investigations performed. Parents must register stillbirth within 42 days.
Subsequent pregnancies: classify as high risk, and manage accordingly.

C: Psychological: ↑ risk of postnatal depression. Infection. Difficulty in establishing labour. DIC if fetus retained >4 weeks (rare before this).

P: Chance of subsequent successful pregnancy depends on cause.

Intrauterine growth restriction

D: Slowing of fetal growth resulting from the presence of a congenital anomaly or acquired circumstance (e.g. infection), so that it does not reach its growth potential.

A:
1 Chromosomal malformation. (Mosaic placenta-chromosome 16)
2 Inadequate supply/placental transfer of nutrients.
3 Congenital.

A/R: **Maternal:** medical problem (hypertensive disorder, diabetes, severe anaemia, hypoxia, antiphospholipid antibodies, other cardiovascular, GI or renal disorders), Rhesus isoimmunization, poor nutrition, drugs (smoking, alcohol, recreational drugs), lower socioeconomic status.
Fetal: transplacental infection (CMV, toxoplasmosis), multiple pregnancy.
Uteroplacental insufficiency: inadequate trophoblastic invasion, antiphospholipid syndrome, diabetes mellitus, sickle cell disease, pre-eclampsia, antepartum haemorrhage.

E: Incidence difficult to confirm because of inaccurate assessment, intraobserver error, maternal constitutional differences, etc.

H: Usually no presenting complaint. ? History of viral illness. At risk: previous baby weighing < 2500 g, stillbirth, neonatal death within first week, known risk factors, multiple pregnancy, vaginal bleed, decreased fetal movement, recurrent UTI.

E: Note maternal constitution. Fundal height < 3 cm below expected size for gestational age (exclude PROM). ? Easily palpable fetal parts (oligohydramnios). ? ↑ Blood pressure (pre-eclampsia)/signs of other medical disorders.

P: Small fetal size. Either symmetrical (normal body proportions) or asymmetrical (reduced abdominal girth comparative to head circumference, secondary to hypoxic circulatory compensation).

I: *Urine*: protein (pre-eclampsia). *Fetal well-being*: fetal movement counts, CTG. *Imaging*: serial ultrasound (fetal growth—2 weekly intervals, fetal abnormality, liquor volume), Doppler study (placental vascular resistance), biophysical profile. *Other*: amniocentesis/cordocentesis (cytology) + karyotype (? genetic defect).

M: **High-risk groups:** more frequent antenatal appointments, serial ultrasound (growth assessment).
Detected IUGR: optimize maternal health (medical conditions, nutrition, stop smoking and other drugs).
Non-compromised fetus: monitor as outpatient (USS, CTG) every 2 weeks.
Compromised fetus: *Mature* (> 34 weeks): consider delivery. *Immature*: inpatient bed rest, intensive fetal surveillance (above investigations), ? low-dose aspirin, ? nitric oxide donors, ? antioxidants, ? oxygen (NB administer steroids if delivery considered < 34 weeks).

C: **Maternal:** complications from causative factors, ↑ breech presentation.
Fetal: intrauterine death, premature delivery, perinatal/neonatal morbidity (birth asphyxia, neonatal hypoglycemia, polycythaemia secondary to hypoxia), perinatal/neonatal mortality, physical/mental handicap, ↑ risk of adult hypertension and diabetes mellitus.

P: Depends on how soon diagnosis is made, premature delivery. Good long-term prognosis for survivors. If congenital/chromosomal abnormality present, development depends on abnormality.

Kallmann's syndrome

D: Isolated GnRH deficiency from the hypothalamus and one or more non-gonadal congenital anomalies, e.g. anosmia.

A: Maldevelopment of neurones in the arcuate nucleus of the hypothalamus.

A/R: Midline facial abnormalities (e.g. cleft palate), urogenital tract abnormalities, red–green colour blindness.

E: Rare.

H: Delayed puberty, primary amenorrhoea, anosmia.

E: Prepubertal (Tanner Stage 0), may be tall as epiphyses fail to fuse because of lack of oestrogen.

P: The neurones are derived embryologically from the olfactory bulb, thus the affected individual also fails to develop a sense of smell.

I: *Bloods:* estradiol, FSH, LH and GH levels. *Others:* Anterior pituitary function tests. Pituitary MRI (exclude tumour).

M: HRT for those not trying to conceive. Pulsatile SC or IV GnRH or IM FSH for those wishing to conceive.

C: Creutzfeldt–Jakob disease (CJD): prior to use of recombinant analogue, GnRH was previously extracted from cadavers resulting in CJD transmission to a small number of patients.

P: Good with correct management.

Lichen sclerosus

D: A chronic, non-neoplastic, inflammatory dermatosis of the vulva.

A: Unknown. ? Autoantibodies to collagen.

A/R: Autoimmune disease (e.g. thyroid disease, IDDM, pernicious anaemia, SLE, primary billiary sclerosis, bullous pemphigoid), vitiligo or family history of autoimmune disease.

E: 1 in 1000, but up to 1 in 30 in elderly patients. Mostly affects postmenopausal women and occasionally prepubertal girls. F > M (10:1).

H: Pruritus vulvae (severe and persistent). Superficial dyspareunia, dysuria, pain and bleeding from affected areas.

E: **Lesions:** usually affect vulva in partial or complete 'figure of eight' manner. Neck and upper back may be affected. May begin as small, white, individual papules, merging to form atrophic, white, 'paper-like' plaques. No invasion of vestibule, vagina or anus.
Pelvic: vulval atrophy, fusion of midline structures, areas of ecchymoses, ulceration, red 'bruised' areas may be mistaken for sexual abuse in the prepubertal girl.
Bimanual: narrowing of introitus may make speculum examination difficult.

P: **Epidermis:** atrophy/thickening/hyperkeratinization.
Dermis: oedema, collagen hyalinization.
Subdermis: lymphocytic infiltration.

I: *Diagnostic:* biopsy of lesion.

M: Local **potent** corticosteroids: clobetasol, β methasone or fluocinolone applied nightly for 1 month, then alternate nights for 1 month and then twice weekly for 1 month. Maintenance treatment when needed.

C: Squamous cell carcinoma of the vulva (5 %). Sexual dysfunction.

P: Chronic condition, usually life long. Childhood presentation has a better prognosis with ∼ 50 % of cases resolving by menarche.

Malposition

D: Refers to the fetal presenting part. Position of the denominator other than occipitoanterior.

A: Uterine contractions are insufficient to flex the fetal head and facilitate rotation to occiptoanterior or pelvic shape/size does not permit rotation leading to occipitoposterior (occiput at 6 o'clock), occipitotransverse (occiput at 3 or 9 o'clock) or oblique (occiput at 10, 2, 4 or 8 o'clock) positions.

A/R: Insufficient uterine contractions, android pelvis, prematurity, abnormal liquor volume, IUD, congenital abnormalities, multiple pregnancies.

E: n/a

H: Incidental diagnosis before labour or via examination during labour; prolonged labour.

E: **General:** ? maternal exhaustion.
Abdominal: lower abdomen appears flattened, limbs palpable, ? high presenting part.
Vaginal: assess station, presentation, position (by examination of the sutures and fontanelles); assess pelvic size; assess cervical dilation.

P: n/a

I: CTG (fetal well-being/frequency, strength and duration of uterine contractions); maternal FBC; group and save if surgery anticipated.

M: **Medical:** oxytocin infusion (augment uterine contractions); epidural (↓ backache); ensure adequate hydration.
Surgical: CS preferable if head two-fifths palpable or cephalopelvic disproportion; otherwise ventouse (to induce flexion and encourage rotation); Kielland's forceps **only** if experienced obstetrician (NB maternal and fetal trauma).
Other: ? manual rotation.

C: **Fetal:** ↑ moulding; fetal distress; sequelae of instrumental delivery.
Maternal: backache (↑ pressure of presenting part on back); bearing down before full cervical dilation (↑ pressure on rectum) →↑ risk perineal tearing.

P: Good. With occipitoposterior 75 % rotate spontaneously to occipitoanterior, others require assisted delivery (20 % deep transverse arrest; 5 % true posterior).

Malpresentation

D: Any presentation whereby the presenting part is not the fetal vertex. Includes breech, face, brow, compound presentations associated with oblique or transverse lies and cord presentations.

A:
1 Obstruction of lower uterine segment.
2 Fetal abnormality.
3 Prematurity.
4 Polyhydramnios.

A/R: **Obstruction:** placenta praevia, pelvic mass, pelvic abnormalities, fibroids, ovarian cysts.
Fetal abnormalities: neural tube defects, hydrocephalus, neuromuscular defects.

E: **Breech:** 1 in 30 at term (1in 4 of premature births).
Transverse: 1 in 200.
Face: 1 in 500.
Brow: 1 in 1000.

H: Asymptomatic, epigastric discomfort (breech).

E: Breech and transverse presentations usually detected antenatally.
Breech: *Abdominal*: palpable head at fundus. *VE during labour*: buttocks or foot felt.
Transverse: *Abdominal*: lower fundal height, abnormal uterine shape (elongated laterally), palpable head laterally (usually to left). *VE during labour*: obstructed labour with limb presenting if neglected.
Face and brow presentations are usually detected during labour.
Face: presenting part high, large amount of head palpable on same side as back: prolonged labour, landmarks of face on VE.
Brow: presenting part high, head fails to engage, bregma at centre of cervix, supraorbital ridges and base of nose felt on VE.

P: n/a

I: USS antenatally to confirm lie and presentation. Breech may be extended (two-thirds) with both legs straight, flexed (both legs bent) or footling (foot is lower than buttock).

M: **Breech:** observe until 37 weeks. If still breech consider ECV (see p. 108). If fails perform ELCS at 39 weeks. Consider vaginal delivery if it is second twin or if mother requests (no maternal/fetal complications, flexed head, not footling and < 4.0 kg). Vaginal delivery requires specific management by experienced staff.
Transverse: admit at 37 weeks in case of ROM (↑ risk cord prolapse), discharge if spontaneous version occurs and persists for > 48 h. If not consider either ECV and amniotomy by senior obstetrician or CS when transverse position stabilizes.
Face: *Mentoanterior position* (90 %): expect long labour with spontaneous delivery. *Mentotransverse position*: rotate to mentoanterior manually, and then forceps delivery. *Mentoposterior*: CS. Warn parents that baby's face may be quite severely distorted because of oedema (subsides within days).
Brow: CS: vaginal delivery is impossible unless fetus converts to face or vertex.

C: **Mother:** ↑ morbidity resulting from CS, uterine rupture (especially transverse), prolonged/obstructed labour, ↑ PPH.
Fetus: ↑ congenital abnormalities, ↑ perinatal mortality (but prematurity contributes significantly to this), ↑ cord prolapse.

P: Depends on cause.

Mendelson's syndrome

D: Destructive pneumonitis occurring as a result of inhalation of acid gastric contents.

A: Regurgitation and aspiration of acidic gastric contents, typically following anaesthesia.

A/R: Anaesthesia (depressed gag reflex), emergency surgery, pregnancy (delayed gastric emptying, ? intra-abdominal pressure), other loss of consciousness, e.g. head injury.

E: n/a

H: Vomiting/regurgitation followed by dyspnoea, cough, pleurisy (if patient not under anaesthesia).

E: Shortness of breath, tachypnoea, wheeze, crackles (on auscultation), cyanosis, tachycardia, pyrexia.

P: Pulmonary inflammation—destruction of alveolar lining, transudation of fluid into alveolar space.

I: *Bloods*: ABG. *Other*: CXR (cloudy opacities, especially lower lobes), pulse oximetry.

M: **Prevention:** preoperative H_2 antagonist, e.g. ranitidine, sodium citrate, aspiration of gastric contents, cricoid pressure with induction of general anaesthetic.
Treatment: tilt patient's head down and turn to one side. Aspirate pharynx. Give 100 % oxygen, aminophylline 5 mg/kg (slow IV), hydrocortisone 500 mg (IV bolus), prophylactic antibiotics, e.g. ampicillin and an aminoglycoside (e.g. gentamicin). Positive pressure ventilation (if needed). Arrange physiotherapy and bronchoscopy with mucus plug aspiration (under general anaesthetic).

C: Pulmonary oedema, secondary bacterial pneumonia, ARDS, death.

P: Mortality 50 %.

Menopause

D: The cessation of normal menstruation. **Climacteric**: symptomatic perimenopausal years.

A: **Climacteric**: decreasing ovarian response to FSH, LH and oestrogen secretion.
Menopause: ovarian failure.
Iatrogenic menopause: removal of the ovaries or uterus/ secondary to radiotherapy or chemotherapy.

E: Universal phenomenon of age. Average age 51 years (UK).
Premature menopause < 40 years (1 % prevalence).

H: Menopause: persistent amenorrhoea (12 months).
Early climacteric features: menstrual irregularity. *Vasomotor symptoms*: hot flushes (flushes and perspiration), night sweats, palpitation, headaches. *Vaginal symptoms*: vaginal dryness and burning, dyspareunia. *Psychological symptoms*: insomnia, poor concentration, lethargy, irritability, ↓ libido, anxiety, depression.
Intermediate climacteric features (2–4 years): breast atrophy, skin changes, hair loss, urinary frequency, incontinence.

E: Breast atrophy, vaginal atrophy, uterine prolapse, thin dry skin.

I: *Bloods*: plasma FSH > 20 IU/L (confirms menopause in ambiguous cases), oestrogen (not as reliable initially).

M: Counselling (changes occurring, general health, diet, lifestyle, HRT), topical oestrogen (vaginal symptoms), HRT (see p. 111), ? clonidine (50–75 mg/ 12 h, for hot flushes).

C: **Long-term complications of oestrogen deficiency**: *Bone*: accelerated bone loss → osteoporosis and pathological fractures. *Cardiovascular*: increased risk of arterial disease, IHD, stroke. *Other*: ↓ pelvic floor muscle tone, ↑ risk of Alzheimer's disease.

Menorrhagia 53

D: Excessive menstrual bleeding, exceeding 80 mL/cycle.

A: Idiopathic; DUB; fibroids; endometrial polyps; endometriosis; adenomyosis; PID; endometrial hyperplasia; endometrial carcinoma; IUD; thyroid and coagulation disorders; psychological disturbance.

A/R: As aetiology.

E: 9–14 % females, common around the menarche as a result of anovulatory cycles.

H: Excessive menstrual bleeding—elicit quantity, duration, timing; ? passage of clots; ? associated with dysmenorrhoea/PMS; ? symptoms associated with underlying cause. *pelvic pain, irregular bleed, dyspareunia, postcoital bleed, intermenstrual, thyroid/clotting disorder*

E: ? Signs of anaemia; abdominal/pelvic examination normal or signs of uterine enlargement associated with fibroids, etc; ? evidence of blood loss; ? tenderness on palpation/cervical excitation/adnexal masses (PID/endometriosis); assess uterine mobility (PID); visualize external genitalia for extrauterine cause of bleeding; ? examine thyroid; ? bruising (clotting disorder).

P: Dependent on aetiology.

I: *Bloods*: Hb (anaemia), platelets (↓ rare cause),? clotting studies (e.g. family history of clotting disorder); serum ferritin; LH : FSH (? PCOS); TFT; USS—pelvic mass, fibroids, etc; Pipelle biopsy (exclude endometrial cancer); hysteroscopy (exclude cancer, visualization of polyps, etc); ? D&C; ? laparoscopy if appropriate (? associated with pelvic mass); cervical cytology.

M: **Conservative:** reassurance; ? weight loss advisable.
Medical: prostaglandin synthetase inhibitors, e.g. mefenamic acid especially with dysmenorrhoea (↓ synthesis endometrial prostaglandins); antifibrinolytics, e.g. tranexamic acid (reduce fibrinolysis in the endometrium); combined OCP (↑ regular endometrial shedding); progestogens (? → secretory changes)/progestogen-containing IUCD (endometrial atrophy); Fe supplementation with anaemia.
Surgical: hysterectomy if appropriate and medical treatment unsatisfactory; ? endometrial ablation techniques using laser or electrocautery, e.g. transcervical resection of the endothelium.

C: Fe deficiency anaemia; social disturbance.

P: Medical treatment often successful; however, intractable cases often necessitate surgical intervention.

DD: Ectopic pregnancy, miscarriage, local causes of bleeding—urethral caruncle, cervical carcinoma/polyps, vaginal/vulval lacerations.

Miscarriage (spontaneous abortion)

D: Fetal death < 24 weeks. Includes threatened (T), inevitable (IE), incomplete (IC), missed (M), septic (S) and recurrent (R) (≥ three consecutive miscarriages).

A: Idiopathic: (25%).
Fetal: up to 50% have either structural, chromosomal or genetic defects.
Placental: abnormal implantation (IUCD, low implantation), ischaemia, abruption.
Uterine: congenital abnormalities, fibroids, cervical incompetence (late miscarriage). (\ bicornuate)
Infection: *Salmonella*, *Listeria*, *Brucella*, CMV, *Campylobacter* sp., BV, rubella, Herpes simplex virus, syphilis.
Maternal disease: SLE, anticardiolipin antibodies, antiphospholipid syndrome, pyrexial infections, von Willebrand's, Wilson's disease. lupus anticoagulant (in isolation)
Endocrine: PCOS, luteal insufficiency.
Poisons: cytotoxic drugs.

A/R: DM (especially ↑ Hb A1c), thyroid disease, ↑ age, multiple pregnancy, smoking, alcohol (mild association).

E: 10–15% of pregnancies will end in a clinically apparent miscarriage, ≤ 50% are subclinical (occur very early on—may be mistaken for heavy period). Minor PV bleeding occurs in early stages in 20–25% of pregnancies.

H: **Early:** PV bleeding/brown discharge, cramping lower abdominal pain. Patient may no longer 'feel' pregnant.
Late: ROM, labour pains.
E **Pelvic:** *T*: PV bleeding, closed cervical os. *IE/IC*: heavy PV bleeding and clots. Open cervical os. *C*: uterus contracted. Closed cervical os. *M*: brown discharge, uterus smaller than expected, closed cervical os. *S*: pyrexia, tachycardia, purulent vaginal blood loss.

P: USS: *T*: viable pregnancy. *IE/IC*: retained products of conception. *C*: empty uterus. *M*: absent FH, collapsed gestational sac. > 16 weeks may see fetal skeleton collapse. *S*: main organisms are: *Escherichia coli*, *Streptococcus* spp and *Staphylococcus aureus*. Infection is usually confined to uterus, but may spread locally or haematologically.

I: **Initial:** *Bloods*: FBC (Hb, WCC), serum β-hCG, clotting, group and save. *Urine*: β-hCG. *Others*: USS.
Recurrent: tailor according to clinical presentation. Consider: *Bloods*: FBC (? Hb), glucose, Hb A1c (diabetic control), antiphospholipid and anticardiolipin antibodies (exclude SLE and antiphospholipid syndrome), clotting (exclude clotting disorders), LH:FSH ratios (exclude endocrine causes). *Others*: HVS, parental/fetal karyotyping, laparoscopy/hysteroscopy.

M: *T*: reassure. 50% will go on to have a successful outcome (90% if > 8 weeks and normal gestational sac and contents seen USS). *IE/IC*: give ergometrine and oxytocin in first trimester, Prostaglandin E2 in second trimester. Supportive therapy (correction of blood loss, analgesia, anti D if Rhesus-negative). Consider curettage if process incomplete. *M*: first trimester: suction evacuation; second trimester PGE2 and oxytocin. *R*: treat any underlying cause if identified, e.g. MacDonald suture (cervical incompetence), low-dose aspirin and SC heparin (SLE/antiphospholipid syndrome). *S*: broad-spectrum antibiotics and curettage.

C: Haemorrhage, infection, DIC, psychological trauma.

P: Majority will subsequently have successful pregnancies.

Multiple pregnancy

D: Pregnancy involving more than one fetus.

A: **Monozygous:** division of fertilized egg (early splitting—separate placentae; late splitting—single placental mass).
Dizygous: fertilization of >1 egg by different sperm (separate placentae).

A/R: Previous history; family history; ovulation induction with clomifene or gonadotrophins; African race; ↑ maternal age.

E: Twins: 1 in 80. Triplets: 1 in 80^2.

H: ? Incidental finding; feeling of abdominal enlargement (if multiparous); hyperemesis (↑ β-hCG); excessive fetal movements.

E: **Abdominal:** large fundal height and ↑ girth (spheroidal abdomen); >1 fetal pole; ↑ fetal parts; >1 fetal heart beat.

P: n/a

I: Confirm by USS.

M: Weekly antenatal visits from early pregnancy (critical time for survival 24–30 weeks). Fe and folate supplements.
Monitor: fetal growth monthly (USS); FBC (anaemia); BP (↑ risk eclampsia); UA (gestational diabetes). Anomaly scan (second trimester). ? Prenatal diagnosis (NB serum screening inaccurate).
Labour: ? induction at 40 weeks (↓ placental insufficiency); continuous fetal heart rate monitoring; ensure availability of anaesthetist; paediatrician present at delivery (↑ asphyxia, especially second twin); vaginal delivery more likely if leading twin cephalic; CS if leading twin breech; CS for higher order births; prophylactic Syntometrine/Syntocinon with birth of the second twin (↑ PPH).

C: **Maternal:** ↑ incidence: hyperemesis, eclampsia, anaemia (↑ plasma volume and fetal Fe requirements), PPH and APH (large placenta), vulval varicosities, diabetes (↑ steroid load), exhaustion and emotional distress associated with upbringing of children, puerperal cardiomyopathy.
Fetal: preterm labour; polyhydramnios; fetofetal tranfusion (placental anastomoses with monochorionicity result in one twin developing polyhydramnios and the other oligohydramnios, one twin also develops anaemia and the other polycythaemia); locking (during labour first twin breech, second vertex, head of first locks with chin of second—rare); ↑ incidence: cord prolapse, malpresentation, perinatal mortality, malformations, IUGR after 28 weeks.

P: Increased fetal risks. Maternal risks minimized with appropriate obstetric care.

Oligohydramnios

D: ↓ Liquor volume with deepest pool < 2 cm on USS.

A: Placental insufficiency, ↓ fetal urine output, ruptured membranes (see p. 70).

A/R: **Fetal:** Urinary tract abnormalities (Potter's syndrome: renal agenesis, posterior urethral valves), chromosomal abnormalities, IUGR, post dates.
Placental: abruption, pre-eclampsia, hypertension, diabetes.
Others: ACE inhibitors, idiopathic.

E: Much less common than polyhydramnios:
< 34 weeks < 1 %
> 34 weeks–term ∼ 2 %
> 41 weeks 10 %.

H: History of complications during pregnancy, leakage of fluid from vagina, ↓ fetal movements.

E: **General:** signs of underlying maternal illness, e.g. ↑ BP, oedema.
Abdomen: ↓ symphysis-fundal height, fetus 'easy to feel'.

P: n/a

I: *Bloods:* glucose. *Urine:* MSU (glycosuria, proteinuria). *Others:* USS with umbilical vessel Doppler, detailed fetal anomaly scan, biophysical profile. Consider CVS (chromosomal abnormalities) depending on gestational age and parental wishes.

M: If ROM manage accordingly (see p. 70).
< **34 weeks:** treat any underlying maternal condition. Admit if any investigations abnormal. Daily CTG, and weekly Doppler and biophysical profile. If evidence of fetal compromise, consider delivery by CS. *Outpatient management*: daily kick chart, weekly Doppler and biophysical profile. Advise mother to come in if fetal movements ↓.
> **34 weeks:** treat any underlying maternal condition. Admit and consider IOL or CS if any investigations abnormal. Outpatient management as above.
> **41 weeks:** IOL.
During labour: continual CTG monitoring, consider amniotransfusion with colloid, ↑ vigilance for cord prolapse.

C: Pulmonary hypoplasia (especially with early presentation), limb deformities (especially flexion deformities, dislocation of hip, club foot), fetal skin → amnion adhesions, IUGR, prematurity, fetal death.
During labour: fetal distress, cord prolapse, ↑ intervention.

P: Poor with early onset ∼ 50 % mortality. Better prognosis in later onset, depending on cause.

Pelvic inflammatory disease

D: Clinical syndrome attributed to infection of one or more internal pelvic organs (endometrium, fallopian tubes, ovaries, parametrium).

A: Routes of infection:
1 Ascending sexually acquired infection (90 %).
2 Childbirth/instrumentation (e.g. TOP).
3 Intraperitoneal spread (e.g. appendicitis).
4 Haematogenous spread (e.g. tuberculosis).
5 Lymphatic dissemination (puerperal infection) + may be complicated by opportunistic bacteria.
Organism: *Chlamydia trachomatis* (50–65 %), gonococcal infection (15–30 %), staphylococcus, streptococcus, *Escherichia coli*, *Streptococcus faecalis*. Often polymicrobial.

A/R: Young, sexually active, multiple partners, previous history, lower socio-economic status, IUCD, early age of first intercourse.
↓ Risk—COC pill (? progesterone thickens cervical mucus), condom use.

E: 1–2 % of sexually active women per year. Peak incidence of at 15–25 years of age.

H: Asymptomatic/pelvic pain (constant dull ache, worsened by movement), dyspareunia, fever, purulent vaginal discharge, irregular menstruation, pelvic mass, RUQ pain (perihepatitis + perihepatic adhesion—Fitz-Hugh–Curtis syndrome).

E: **General:** pyrexia, tachycardia.
Bimanual: bilateral suprapubic tenderness, ? adnexal tenderness, cervical excitation, ? palpable mass.
Abdominal: abdominal muscle spasm, rigidity, ? rebound tenderness (if peritonitis).

P: Infection and inflammation of one or more pelvic organs ± tissue scarring and adhesions.

I: *Bloods*: FBC (? neutrophilia), U&E, ESR, culture (if severe pyrexia), ? CRP. *Urine*: MSU and culture. *Other*: endocervical swab (for *Chlamydia*, ELISA, *Neisseria gonorrhoea* and anaerobe culture); urethral and cervical swabs (culture and antibiotic sensitivity). *Imaging*: abdominal ultrasound (? abcess, pyosalpinx, etc); laparoscopy (red, swollen fallopian tubes, ? pus, ? abcess)/transvaginal ultrasound + endometrial sample (if pelvic mass/treatment failure/doubt of diagnosis).

M: **Medical:** bed rest, hospital admission (severe cases), adequate fluids, correct electrolytes, analgesia (NSAIDs, opiates), antibiotics (start broad-spectrum antibiotics, e.g. doxycycline + metronidazole/azithromycin +/− a penicillin before culture results).
Surgical: conservative surgery e.g. abcess drainage, lavage (failed drug treatment/pelvic mass).
Other: trace and treat contacts, follow-up (∼ 1 week), advise re: fertility, ? risk ectopic pregnancy.

C: **Chronic infection:** pelvic abscess, pyosalpinx, hydrosalpinx.
Tissue scarring and adhesions: tubal blockage, infertility, increased risk of ectopic pregnancy, Asherman's syndrome.

P: **Recurrence:** 30 % (1 year).
Ectopic: 7–10-fold increased risk.
Infertility: 15–20 % increases to > 50 % after 2–3 recurrences.

Placental abruption

D: Partial or complete separation of a normally implanted placenta prior to delivery of fetus.

A: 95% unknown. Others: trauma (e.g. ECV, road accident, blow to uterus), short cord, sudden reduction in uterine size (e.g. ROM in polyhydramnios).

A/R: Hypertension (pre-eclampsia, essential), previous history, ↑ age, polyhydramnios, multiple pregnancy, clotting disorders, fibroids, smoking, ↑ AFP in absence of fetal abnormality.

E: 1 in 200.

H: Abdominal/back pain (constant, severe, ↑ over specific uterine area). Uterine contractions. Vaginal bleeding (dark, red, heavy. Absent if concealed abruption). Syncope.

E: **General:** shock—may be out of proportion to blood loss. DIC—widespread bleeding, petechia.
Abdomen: Uterus: tender, contracted, 'woody', hard. Difficulty in feeling fetus and obtaining fetal heart.
Pelvic: VE **never** performed until placenta praevia excluded.

P: Vicious cycle established: bleeding from maternal venous sinus results in retroplacental clot which detaches part of placenta, causing further bleeding which spreads from site of original clot and further detachment of placenta. The blood may:
1 track down between myometrium and membranes;
2 enter the amniotic fluid (bloodstained);
3 track into the myometrium (→ bruised, indurated appearance of uterus on CS—*Couvelaire uterus*).
The latter two may result in a concealed abruption (25%), especially if the edges of the placenta or membranes remain attached to uterus, or fetal head closely applied to lower uterine segment. Thromboplastins from damaged placenta and ↑ consumption of clotting factors and platelets can cause DIC.

I: *Bloods:* FBC (↓ Hb), clotting, U&E, cross-match 6 units, Kleihauer test (maternal–fetal haemorrhage). *Others*: CTG (establish fetal viability), USS (exclude placenta praevia).

M: **Basic:** admit and resuscitate. Correct coagulation defects (FFP and platelets). Catheterize—monitor urine output. Analgesia (opiate)—avoid epidural because of risk of coagulopathy. Anti D to Rhesus-negative women.
Delivery: *Mild* (<500 mL blood loss, no maternal/fetal complications, no retroplacental clots on USS): <37 weeks—give steroids and observe for 5 days; discharge if no further bleeding. >37 weeks—IOL or CS. *Moderate/severe*: If fetus alive and distressed—urgent CS. If fetus alive and not distressed—amniotomy and vaginal delivery, *or* CS. If fetus dead—amniotomy and vaginal delivery. CS if severe haemorrhage.
Post-partum: ↑ observation for PPH.

C: DIC, renal failure, maternal/fetal death, Sheehan's syndrome, post-partum haemorrhage.

P: Mortality: fetal 30%, maternal 0.5%.

Placenta praevia

D: Either part or all of the placenta is implanted into the lower uterine segment.

A: Unknown. Hypotheses include late implantation of blastocyst, simple accident of nature or damaged endometrium preventing implantation.

A/R: Multiparity, ↑ age, multiple pregnancy, uterine damage (e.g. from previous surgery).

E: 0.5 % of all pregnancies at term. Accounts for 20 % of cases of APH.

H: Three typical presentations:
1 **APH**: usually recurrent painless haemorrhages beginning in third trimester (60 % = 36 weeks, 30 % at 32–36 weeks and 10 % < 32 weeks) and ↑ in severity with each bleed.
2 **Fetal malpresentation**: low-lying placenta prevents fetal turning/head engagement.
3 **Detected on routine USS**.

E: APH: *General*: shock. *Abdomen*: uterus soft and non-tender. High head/malpresentation. VE must **never** be performed in suspected placenta praevia.

P: Classified as:
1 *Minor (previously grades I and II)*: placenta on lower segment, but does not cover internal os.
2 *Major (previously grades III and IV)*: placenta either partially (grade III) or completely covers internal os (grade IV).
Bleeding occurs as a result of cervical dilation, or ↑ size of lower uterine segment resulting in shearing forces to the placental attachment.

I: APH: *Bloods*: FBC, U&E, clotting, cross-match. *Others*: USS, CTG (assess fetal well-being).
Malpresentation/routine USS: if low-lying placenta diagnosed early on in pregnancy, repeat USS at 32 and 36 weeks as placenta may 'rise' up as a result of formation of lower uterine segment. ~ 10 % of low-lying placentas diagnosed early on will be praevia at term.

M: APH: *Severe*: resuscitate and senior person should deliver fetus immediately by CS. *Less severe*:
1 admit and assess maternal and fetal well-being and severity of placenta praevia;
2 give anti D to Rhesus-negative women;
3 corticosteroids until 34 weeks (↑ fetal lung maturity);
4 if possible wait until 39 weeks for delivery by CS. Vaginal delivery may only be attempted if fetal head is below placental edge and grade of praevia is minor.
No APH: consider routine admission at 32 weeks if major. Manage as above.

C: APH, ↑ risk of haemorrhage during CS and PPH (vessels in lower uterine segment do not contract as well as in other areas of uterus).

P: If managed well, maternal and perinatal mortality is low.

Polyhydramnios

D: Abnormally increased amniotic fluid volume.

A: 1 *Idiopathic.*
2 ↑ *Fetal urine output*: macrosomia, twin–twin transfusion syndrome (recipient twin), tumour, hydrops fetalis.
3 ↓ *Fetal GI absorption*: gastroschisis, exomphalos, oesophageal atresia, duodenal atresia, Hirschsprung's disease.
4 ↓ *Fetal swallowing*: anencephaly, spina bifida, facial tumour, macroglossia, myotonic dystrophy.
5 ↑ *Secretion of amniotic fluid by large placenta*: diabetes, multiple pregnancy.

A/R: Diabetes (20 %), congenital fetal abnormality (5 %), multiple pregnancy.

E: 1 % of pregnancies.

H: May present acutely or chronically. Usually onset is gradual and in third trimester.
Acute: severe abdominal pain, oesophageal reflux, worsening haemorrhoids/varicose veins, 'bursting' feeling, dyspnoea, vomiting.
Chronic: asymptomatic, abdomen is larger than expected, ↑ fetal movements, and symptoms as for acute.

E: General: peripheral oedema, varices.
Abdomen: uterus large for dates, fetus difficult to feel, FH difficult to hear, fluid thrill. *Acute*: striae, glazed and oedematous abdominal skin, tense and tender uterus.

P: Normal amniotic fluid volume = 500–1500 mL. Symptoms and signs are produced when volume > 2L and result from ↑ uterine size and weight.

I: *Blood*: Rhesus status. *Others*: USS (confirm ↑ amniotic fluid volume as deepest pool > 10 cm and exclude multiple pregnancy and fetal abnormalities), biophysical profile (assess fetal well-being), GTT (exclude diabetes).

M: Treat only symptomatic cases. If USS reveals a gross fetal abnormality parents must be counselled.
1 Treat underlying cause if identified, e.g. improved control of diabetes.
2 If minor—night time sedation to relieve discomfort.
3 Consider amniocentesis (remove ∼ 500 mL fluid) or indometacin (↓ fetal urine output). Successful in ∼ 50 % cases, but ↑ risk of PDA closure and renal impairment.
4 ↑ Fetal surveillance.

C: Malpresentation, stillbirth, placental abruption, cord prolapse, APH, PPH, ↑ CS rate.

P: Depends on underlying cause. An identifiable cause cannot be found in 60 % of cases.

Polycystic ovarian syndrome

D: Also Stein–Levanthal syndrome. A persistent anovulatory state characterized by androgen excess, continuing oestrogenization, elevated serum LH with low FSH.

A: Unknown. Ovarian androgen hypersecretion increases pituitary sensitivity to GnRH. ? Adrenal hyperandrogenism in some. Resultant increase in LH secretion causes further androgen secretion. Vicious cycle of ovarian, adrenal, hypothalamo-pituitary malfunction → disrupts hormone balance. ? Inherited/acquired insulin resistance (insulin; gonadotrophic, influences LH and FSH → ovarian disorder).

A/R: Family history.

E: 75 % incidence in those with fertility problems or ovulatory problems. 5–10 % premenopausal women.

H: Amenorrhoea; DUB; obesity; hirsutism; virilization; recurrent miscarriage; failure to conceive; acne.

E: ? Obesity; ? hirsutism; examination often entirely normal.

P: Ovaries are enlarged, show multiple, small, follicular cysts (derived from ovarian follicles and lined by granulosa cells) without developing a dominant follicle, particularly around periphery; thickening of the ovarian stroma; ? ↑ oestrogen levels → endometrial hyperplasia.

I: Serum LH ↑; serum FSH ↔; →↑ LH:FSH ratio (>3:1); ↑ oestrogen; ? ↑ testosterone; ↓ steroid hormone binding protein; ? ↑ PRL; positive progestogen challenge; USS—enlarged ovaries with typical 'icing sugar' capsule; ? laparoscopy (rule out pelvic pathology).

M: Medical: OCP/progestogen (for unopposed oestrogenization, to induce regular bleeds). ? OCP preparation with antiandrogen cyproterone acetate—Dianette (hirsutism). ? anti-oestrogen clomifene (subfertility). ? Use of metformin for metabolic and endocrine abnormalities, ↓ weight and ↑ menstrual cyclicity (cf. insulin resistance).
Surgical: hysterectomy last resort for menstrual problems. Laparoscopic ovarian surgery, e.g. wedge resection/laser drilling (subfertility).
Other: maintenance of normal body weight—(prevent insulin resistance); dietary/lifestyle changes; cosmetic options for hirsutism.

C: Hirsutism, psychological sequelae, risk of endometrial cancer (unopposed oestrogenization); ↑ risk cardiovascular disease; subfertility; recurrent miscarriage.

P: With treatment many symptoms can be controlled although hirsutism may be difficult to overcome. Infertility may require substantial attention.

Polyp: cervical and endometrial

D: Cervical (C): local proliferation of cervical mucosa.
Endometrial (E): local proliferation of endometrial glands.

A: C, local inflammation; E, ↑ oestrogen levels.

A/R: C: recurrent genitourinary infections, e.g. thrush, bacterial vaginosis.
E: unopposed oestrogen therapy, climateric phase, obesity, PCOS, tamoxifen therapy, oestrogen-secreting tumours.

E: C: 5 % of women. Most common > 40 years.
E: uncommon < 30 years. Present in 10 % women > 50 years.

H: C: asymptomatic, PCB, IMB, PMB, menorrhagia, chronic vaginal discharge (clear, non-offensive).
E: asymptomatic, PMB, IMB, menorrhagia.

E: C: *Speculum*: may see polyp protruding through external os. Bleeds easily.
E: usually unremarkable.

P: C: *Macro*: red, small (usually < 1 cm), soft growth. Usually pedunculated. *Micro*: Proliferation of columnar epithelium of the endocervical canal. Contain dilated, mucus-secreting endocervical glands. Hallmarks of inflammation and squamous metaplasia are commonly present.
E: *Macro*: most commonly located in uterine fundus, seen as a dark red, velvety, oval lesion. May be single or multiple. Usually sessile. Vary in size from 0.5 to 3 cm. *Micro*: two patterns identified. Most frequent is a histological appearance of cystic hyperplasia (endometrial glands of varying size, proliferative changes). The other is functional, i.e. histologically the lesion is the same as the surrounding normal endometrium.

I: *Bloods*: FBC (↓ Hb). *Others*: cervical smear (exclude CIN/malignancy), HVS (exclude infection), hysteroscopy (diagnostic), USS (measure endometrial thickness).

M: Medical: treat anaemia if present.
Surgical: polypectomy at hysteroscopy—loop cutting diathermy or avulsion with forceps.

C: Local (infection, torsion or necrosis of tip). Anaemia. Haemorrhage following surgical removal. Malignant change (rare).

P: Surgical removal cures most cases.

Post-coital bleeding

D: Vaginal bleeding following intercourse that is not associated with menstruation.

A: Cervical carcinoma, cervical eversion/erosion, cervical polyps, cervicitis, trauma, infection (*Chlamydia, Trichomonas*), pregnancy (e.g. placenta praevia).

A/R: Cervical carcinoma (see p. 16), cervical eversion/erosion (see p. 22), cervical polyps (see p. 62), cervicitis (see p. 24), trauma: vigorous intercourse, recent smear/colposcopy.

E: Relatively common.

H: May give history of abnormal smears or evidence of infection (e.g. abnormal discharge).

E: **Pelvic:** *Inspection*: vaginal discharge. *Speculum*: ectopy/ectropian, polyps, friability, ulcerations.

P: Absence of healthy squamous cell epithelium predisposes to bleeding with mild trauma, i.e. intercourse.

I: Cervical smear, endocervical and HVS for infection, colposcopy (if persistent PCB). If pregnant exclude causes of APH, e.g. placenta praevia.

M: Manage according to results of investigation. Aci-Jel (acetic acid) may be used to enhance metaplasia of columnar epithelium to squamous epithelium.

C: n/a

P: Most cases of PCB are benign in origin and are easily treated.

Postmenopausal bleeding

D: Vaginal bleeding occurring ≥ 6 months after menopause.

A: Non-pathological: withdrawal bleeding from HRT.
Pathological: *Uterus*: carcinoma, hyperplasia (may be atypical), polyps. *Ovaries*: oestrogen secreting tumour. *Vagina*: **atrophic vaginitis** (by far the most common cause), carcinoma, foreign body, e.g. shelf/ring pessary. *Vulva*: carcinoma. *Cervix*: carcimona, cervicitis, polyps.

A/R: Non-pathological: see p. 114.
Pathological: *Uterus*: carcinoma (see p. 17), hyperplasia (see p. 17), polyps (see p. 62). *Ovaries*: tumour (see p. 18). *Vagina*: atrophic vaginitis (see p. 9), foreign body: prolapse (may require use of pessary). *Vulva*: carcinoma (see pp. 19, 94). *Cervix*: carcinoma (see pp. 16, 23), cervicitis (see p. 24), polyps (see p. 62).

E: Relatively common.

H: Withdrawal bleeding presents with regular cyclical bleeding. Pathological causes usually present with isolated incidence of PMB, or recurrent episodes of irregular PMB. Other symptoms depend on cause, e.g. dyspareunia with atrophic vaginitis.

E: Depends on cause.
Pelvic: *Inspection*: vaginal atrophy. *Bimanual*: ↑ uterine size (uterine hyperplasia/carcinoma), pelvic mass (ovarian tumour). *Sims*: uterine prolapse (cervicitis), foreign body. *Cusco*: ulcerated, friable cervix (carcinoma, chronic cervicitis), polyps.

P: n/a

I: *Bloods*: FBC (↓ Hb). *Others*: cervical smear, pelvic USS (uterine thickness), hysteroscopy and endometrial biopsy.

M: Full history to assess risk factors for malignancy and to exclude withdrawal bleeding. Investigate as above to exclude carcinoma. Treat underlying cause.

C: Anaemia, complications from hysteroscopy (see p. 113).

P: Approximiately 5% of women presenting with PMB will have cancer (uterine carcinoma being the most common). Benign causes are usually easily treated.

Postnatal blues

D: Self-limiting alteration of emotional state that occurs in the early postnatal period.

A: Unclear. Hormonal basis? (postnatal decrease in progesterone, oestrogen, sodium?)/reaction to the major event of childbirth.

A/R: PMS, social/marital problems.
Prolonged blues: post-partum pyrexia, anaemia, inadequate sleep, delayed healing of episiotomy/caesarean wound, delay in establishing breastfeeding.

E: 50–70 % of women.

H: Onset commonly 3–5 days post-partum. Emotional lability, crying (without cause), sadness, irritability, sleep disturbance, poor concentration, headaches, feeling vulnerable, disproportionate fear of inability to cope with baby.

E: No physical signs.

P: No identifiable pathology.

I: No investigations required.

M: **Antenatal:** education about 'blues' (helpful).
Postnatal: reassurance, ? support groups.

C: Postnatal depression (↑ risk if persists for longer than 2 weeks)/psychosis.

P: Good. Self-limiting (usually lasts less than 1 week, may persist for 1 month, more than one episode may occur).

Postnatal depression

D: Disorder of emotion, involving a pervasive lowering of mood that is initiated in the postnatal period.

A: Appears to be predominantly social factors.

A/R: Family/personal history of depression (especially post-partum). Marital conflict, lack of confiding relationships. Adverse life event before/during pregnancy, complicated pregnancy. Ambivalent to motherhood. Single, young. Chronic life difficulties. Lack of sleep, fatigue.

E: 10–15 % of new mothers.

H: Onset within 6 weeks post-partum. Low mood (worse in the morning), early morning waking, decreased appetite, feelings of guilt and inadequacy with baby, poor concentration, anhedonia (loss of ability to feel enjoyment), anxiety (excess anxiety about baby's health and safety), irritability, suicidal ideation (rare).

E: No abnormal signs.

P: No identifiable pathology.

I: No investigations required.

M: Detection: assess mother for depression at 6 weeks postnatal check.
Treatment: depends on patient severity, circumstance and preference.
Options: psychotherapy (supportive/cognitive), marital therapy, counselling, oral antidepressants (slight risk if breastfeeding), NB evidence for use of daily oestrogen, support groups.

C: Physical morbidity, suicide/infanticide, prolonged depression, post-partum psychosis, persistent abnormality of mother–child interaction, psychiatric morbidity of child, marital breakdown.

P: 50 % remain depressed after 1 year. Good outcome with treatment. 50 % recurrence in subsequent pregnancies.

Post-partum haemorrhage

D: **Primary PPH:** blood loss > 500 mL within 24 h of delivery.
Secondary PPH: blood loss > 500 mL 24 h → 6 weeks after delivery.

A: **Primary (P):** ~80 % caused by uterine atony and/or retained placenta (full/part/accessory lobe). Remainder caused by genital tract trauma (~20 %), e.g. perineal, vaginal or cervical tear, episiotomy, coagulation disorders (DIC, idiopathic thrombocytopaenic purpura, von Willebrand's disease), placenta accreta (chorionic villi invade deep into myometrium preventing complete separation after delivery), uterine inversion.
Secondary (S): endometritis, poor epithelialization of placental bed, retained placental parts, choriocarcinoma (rare).

A/R: P: Overdistension of uterus (multiple pregnancy, polyhydramnios), multiparity, fibroids, placenta praevia, history of APH, previous history of PPH, prolonged labour, passive management of third stage, operative/instrumental delivery.
S: See risk factors for individual causes.

E: P: 4 % following passive management of third stage, 1 % following active management.
S: < 1 %.

H: P: Sudden onset PV bleeding after delivery.
S: PV bleeding. Labour-like pains. Symptoms of underlying infection, e.g. pyrexia.

E: P: *General*: shock. *Abdomen*: enlarged, uncontracted, 'boggy' uterus (atony). *Pelvic inspection*: genital tract trauma. *Bimanual*: uterine inversion.
S: *Abdomen*: enlarged uterus. *Pelvic bimanual*: tender uterus, open internal cervical os.

P: n/a

I: P: *Bloods:* FBC (↓ Hb), U&E, clotting, cross-match 6 units.
S: As for primary if severe. In addition HVS (infection) and USS (retained placental parts). Histological examination of evacuated tissue (exclude choriocarcinoma).

M: P: *Resuscitate*: (summon extra help, gain venous access (= two large-bore cannulae), catheterize and set up CVP, 20 mL blood for Ix, replace lost fluid with colloid or O-negative blood until cross-matched blood arrives).
Identify and stop bleeding:
1 *Placenta separated, but not delivered*: deliver placenta by Brandt–Andrews method (left hand over lower abdomen, just above pubic symphysis, pushing gently upwards whilst traction is applied to umbilical cord) and rub up contraction. If still bleeding, give 0.25 mg ergometrine IV and consider bimanual compression.
2 *Not separated*: manual removal under GA, then bimanual compression.
3 *If placenta delivered and uterus soft and uncontracted*: rub up contraction and give 0.5 mg IV syntometrine.
4 *If placenta delivered and uterus firm and contracted*: suspect genital tract and manage as appropriate (e.g. suturing).
If bleeding continues despite above treatment:
1 Consider carboprost (PGF$_{2\alpha}$) 250 μg into myometrium.
2 Surgery (uterine artery embolization, B Lynch suture, hysterectomy as very last resort).   ↳ internal iliac a.
S: Resuscitate if severe.
Give ergotamine IM, antibiotics and consider ERPC if USS detects clots or placental parts or bleeding continues.

Post-partum haemorrhage continued

- **C:** Shock, death, DIC, multiorgan failure, ARDS, Sheehan's syndrome (rare—see p. 80), complications of massive blood transfusion.
- **P:** Good if specialist obstetric care available. Remains major cause of maternal mortality in developing world.

Coagulation defects of DIC : fresh frozen plasma or cryoprecipitate.

Pre-eclampsia

D: Hypertension with proteinuria developing during pregnancy, labour or puerperium.

A: Genetic predisposition; abnormal placentation/placental ischaemia; abnormal prostaglandin synthesis/balance; defective bioavailability of nitric oxide.

A/R: Primigravidae; previous history; pre-existing essential hypertension; family history (mother/sister); diabetes; autoimmune disease; renal disease; extremes of reproductive age; multiple pregnancy; molar pregnancy.

E: 3 % of primigravidae.

H: Often asymptomatic; hypertension often detected on routine examination; later: oedema, frontal headache, visual symptoms (raised ICP), oliguria (renal failure), abdominal pain (distension hepatic capsule).

E: General: ↑ BP (two or more diastolic readings of 90 mmHg or an isolated reading of 110 mmHg); **oedema** (especially fingers, facial); **Neurological: papilloedema; hyper-reflexia/clonus** (cerebral oedema).
Respiratory system: ↓ air entry, crepitations (pulmonary oedema); **abdominal palpation:** small fundus (IUGR/oligohydramnios); ? RUQ tenderness.

P: Multisystemic involvement of organs. Reflects endothelial damage (↑ permeability), activation of coagulation cascade.

I: *Bloods*: FBC ↑ PCV, ↓ platelets; coagulation screen; serum uric acid; blood film-haemolysis; LFT: deranged, hypoalbuminaemia; U&E: renal function. *Urine*: urinalysis/MSU–proteinuria, exclude UTI; 24-h urine—proteinuria (> 0.3 g protein in 24 h), ? Vanillylmandelic acid (exclude phaeochromocytoma). *Fetal well-being*: USS/biophysical profile (IUGR, fetal condition); Doppler blood flow studies.

M: Cured only by delivery of fetus and placenta.
> 36 weeks/severe pre-eclampsia: delivery by IOL or LSCS respectively.
< 36 weeks: conservative treatment to prolong pregnancy subject to continuous fetal and maternal monitoring. *Antihypertensives* (methyldopa, nifedipine, hydralazine, labetalol): seizure prophylaxis (magnesium sulphate until 48 h post-partum). *Monitor*: fetal well-being (CTG, USS, Doppler), maternal BP, fluid balance, proteinuria, serum urate, U&E, FBC, clotting, O_2 sats, blood pressure. *Administer*: corticosteroids (fetal lung maturation) if delivery anticipated.

C: Fetal: IUGR, oligohydramnios; death; sequelae of prematurity.
Maternal: multiple organ failure; cerebral haemorrhage; pulmonary oedema; ARDS; hepatic capsule rupture; HELLP; renal failure; DIC, retinal detachment (very rare).

P: Generally good, although 10–15 % recurrence in subsequent pregnancies.

Prelabour rupture of membranes

D: Rupture of fetal membranes prior to onset of established labour.

A: Trauma, e.g. amniocentesis, ? ↓ collagen ? infection (bacterial growth → ↑ pH → weakening of mucosal plug and membrane breakdown. Production of phospholipase A_2 →↑ prostaglandin release → cervical ripening).

A/R: Genital tract infection (especially *Neisseria gonorrhoea*, Group B streptococcus, *Chlamydia trachomatis*, TV, BV, *Escherichia coli* and mycoplasma), chorioamnionitis, placental abruption, UTI, multiple pregnancy, polyhydramnios and cervical incompetence.

E: 2–3 % of pregnancies. Accounts for 50 % of premature deliveries and 10 % of perinatal deaths.

H: A gush of fluid from the vagina followed by continuous trickle. May be accompanied by the onset of uterine contractions shortly after.

E: **General:** signs of infection (tachycardia, pyrexia, hypotension).
Speculum: fluid draining from cervical os. The os may be dilated. Pooling of fluid in posterior fornix. Purulent vaginal discharge (infection).

P: n/a

I: **Diagnostic:** If in doubt test sample of fluid for:
1 *pH*: use Nitrazine stick. Turns dark blue with ? pH (suggestive of amniotic fluid which is alkaline). Beware of false-positives (semen, infection). *(Usually overwe)*
2 *Protein*: absent in urine.
3 *Ferning*: amniotic fluid ferns on a glass slide.
USS to estimate remaining liquor volume.
Exclude infection: *Bloods*: FBC (↑ WCC) ESR, CRP. *Urine*: MSU. *Others*: HVS.

M: Evaluate for signs of infection.
Induce labour if:
1 > 36 weeks: risk of infection > benefit of further maturation) or;
2 *signs of infection*: if infection present give broad-spectrum antibiotics.
If < 36 weeks and no signs of infection:
1 Hospitalize (minimum 10 days).
2 Maternal corticosteroids (dexamethasone IM) to promote fetal lung maturity if < 34 weeks.
3 Monitor for signs of infection and assess fetal well-being (daily CTG, fortnightly USS). Minimize risk of infection, e.g. avoid VE. Use of prophylactic antibiotics has been shown to delay the onset of labour.
4 If infection occurs, give broad-spectrum antibiotics and arrange immediate delivery. *(erythromycin)*
5 Allow labour to continue if it begins spontaneously. Tocolytics considered if transferring to another unit, or to allow 48 h for steroids to take effect.

C: **Ascending infection:** endometritis, septicaemia, neonatal pneumonia.
Oligohydramnios: pulmonary hypoplasia, Potter's syndrome (>50 % affected if < 20 weeks. Lethal condition characterized by pulmonary hypoplasia and limb deformities), positional foot deformities, congenital dislocation of hip, malpresentation, cord compression, cord prolapse.
Prematurity.

P: Spontaneous labour occurs within 24 h in > 80 % and 48 h in > 90 % if > 36 weeks. If < 28 weeks mean time between ROM and delivery is 4 weeks.

Premenstrual syndrome

D: Symptoms arising a week or two before the menstrual period and resolving within a week of its onset, severe enough to cause disturbance to daily living.

A: Unknown: ? abnormal progesterone metabolism → anxiety-inducing pregnenolone instead of allopregnanolone; ? involvement of serotonin and ovarian function → central nervous system biochemistry; ? psychological element.

A/R: Age > 30 years; life stresses; psychiatric morbidity; menstrual disorders; postnatal depression.

E: Mostly women > 30 years. 3 % severe enough to cause disruption to daily activities.

H: Symptoms 7–14 days before the menstrual period; ? relieved by menstruation; variable symptoms including lower abdomen tenderness; backache; mastalgia; bloated sensation; headache; depression; emotional lability.

E: No abnormalities found on pelvic, abdominal or breast examination.

P: n/a

I: *Bloods*: FBC (exclude anaemia). *USS/laparoscopy*: if clinical suspicion of pelvic pathology. *Other*: 3 months prospective menstrual charting.

M: Medical: combined OCP (suppress ovulation); progestogens (redress balance), oestrogen implants/patches with progestogens (suppression of ovarian cycle); prostaglandin synthetase inhibitors (mefenamic acid 12 days before onset of period); antidepressants if appropriate (SSRIs); ? GnRH analogues (only short-term because side-effects); ? bromocriptine/ oil of evening primrose/danazol (mastalgia); ? diuretics (fluid retention); vitamin B_6 (co-factor for neurotransmitters but little evidence). Only GnRH analogues and antidepressants appear to be evidence based.
Surgical: hysterectomy and oophorectomy considered in exceptional circumstances on patient request.
Other: psychosocial intervention if appropriate; reassurance; diaries, e.g. 3 months prospective menstrual charting; anecdotal evidence →↑ exercise and dietary changes including reduction in chocolate and caffeine.

C: Psychological sequelae; disruption of daily life; interference with relationships.

P: May constitute a long-term problem.

Preterm labour

D: Onset of labour before 37 weeks of gestation completed. Labour defined as >2 cm cervical dilatation in presence of painful, regular contractions.

A: Uncertain mechanism of onset, see A/R.

A/R: Idiopathic, multiple pregnancy, polyhydramnios, PROM (local prostaglandin release), previous preterm labour, infection (chorioamnionitis, urinary tract, genital tract especially bacterial vaginosis, other), systemic disorder (diabetes mellitus, hypertension), placental abruption, placenta praevia, uterine malformation, cervical incompetence, APH (irritation of the myometrium), fetal malformation, fetal death, maternal pyrexia.

E: 6% of pregnancies before 37 weeks, 2% of pregnancies before 34 weeks.

H: Gestational period < 36 weeks, labour—1–2 regular painful uterine contractions (each lasting for 30 s) in 10 min, persisting for 60 min ± rupture of membranes, backache, ↓ fetal movement, ↑ vaginal discharge, vaginal bleed.

E: General: ? tachycardia/mild pyrexia/signs of systemic disorder.
VE: cervix dilated (> 2.0 cm), cervix effaced (> 75%), intact/ruptured membranes, repeat after 2 h (change?).
Obstetric assessment of abdomen: palpable contractions.

P: Not proven, theories include: nitric oxide–prostaglandin balance disturbance, cervix as the initiator, infection (? bacteria produce proteolytic enzymes which attack membranes). NB. Regular uterine contractions are normal during pregnancy, and are known as Braxton–Hicks contractions when they become palpable after 30th week of pregnancy.

I: *Bloods*: FBC, ESR, culture (if infection suspected). *Urine*: MSU and culture. *Fetal assessment*: CTG, amniocentesis/cordocentesis (infection), transvaginal ultrasound (predictor of preterm delivery). *Other*: HVS (infection).

M: Dependent on gestation length and stage of labour.
General: observation and CTG monitoring, adequate hydration, appropriate antibiotics (if infection suspected/rupture of membranes), adequate analgesia, steroids (IM/PO), e.g. dexamethasone, betamethasone (if < 34 weeks aids fetal lung maturation →↓ respiratory distress syndrome).
High risk: transfer (if neonatal intensive care facilities unavailable), cervical cerclage (? cervical incompetence suspected).
Tocolytics (↓ success if cervix > 3 cm dilated, caution with APH/SRM, acute use to stop uterine contractions allows transfer/steroid action): β-sympathomimetics, e.g. ritodrine, salbutamol (β2 agonist → smooth muscle relaxation), indomethacin (↓ prostaglandins), Ca^{2+} channel blockers (smooth muscle relaxation), oxytocin receptor antagonists (atosiban).
Delivery: avoid trauma and rupture of membranes.

C: Neonatal death, morbidity (especially respiratory distress syndrome, intraventricular haemorrhage), handicap/developmental abnormality (cerebral palsy, visual/hearing deficit, emotional disturbance, social maladjustment).

P: 24 weeks: 30% survival, 40% handicap; 27 weeks: 80% survival, < 10% handicap. Accounts for 20% of perinatal mortality.

Prolactinoma

D: Prolactin-secreting adenoma of anterior pituitary gland.

A: Unknown.

A/R: MEN type 1, pre-menstrual syndrome, headache.

E: Peak onset 25–35 years. Accounts for up to 50 % of cases of prolactinaemia if PRL > 1000 mU/L.

H: Galactorrhoea, oligomenorrhoea or secondary amenorrhoea, infertility, ↓ libido, headache, visual disturbance. Onset may be in pregnancy when adenoma may ↑ in size (50 % of macroadenomas and 10 % of microadenomas become symptomatic in pregnancy).

E: **Breast:** galactorrhoea, prominent Montgomery tubercles.
Neurological: bitemporal hemianopia.
Pelvic: normal.

P: Classified as either microadenoma (< 10 mm) or macroadenoma (> 10 mm). Arise in the lower lateral wings of the anterior pituitary from lactotrophs as a soft, discrete mass consisting of a pseudocapsule of compressed tissue. Symptoms arise partly because of secretion of large quantities of prolactin. The high prolactin stimulates lactation and has a negative feedback effect on LH production which in turn suppresses the rest of the menstrual cycle.

I: *Bloods*: serum PRL: > 600 mU/L for microadenomas and significantly higher levels for macroadenomas often > 8000 mU/L. Three measurements required (PRL release is pulsatile and stress can ↑ prolactin levels). Serum T4 (hyperthyroidism commonly co-exists), short Synacthen test. *Others*: pituitary MRI/CT, visual field test with Goldman perimetry, SXR (erosion of clinoid process and sella turcica, especially with macroadenomas).

M: Treat all macroadenomas and symptomatic microadenomas.
Medical: *Bromocriptine*: dopamine (DA) agonist. Effective in 90 %. Start at 1.25 mg/day, increasing to a maximum of 30 mg/day. *Cabergoline*: long-acting DA agonist. Used in those resistant to bromocriptine. Fewer side-effects. Start at 0.25 mg 2 × week, increasing to maximum of 1 mg 2 × week. CI in pregnancy so must switch to bromocriptine 1 month before conception. *Quinagolid*: used if above fail. Long-acting DA agonist. Costs restrict use.
Surgical: transphenoidal selective adenectomy. Used for large tumours with suprasellar and frontal extension or non-functioning macroadenomas. Follow-up with radiotherapy.

C: Tumour expansion (macro = 25 %, micro = 1–5 % risk) resulting in worsening bitemporal hemianopia or panhypopituitarism, recurrence following surgery (macro = 90 %, micro = 40 %). Osteoporosis, side-effects of drugs (GI disturbance, dizziness, syncope, postural hypotension, cold peripheries, psychosis).

P: 1 in 3 of adenomas regress spontaneously.

Prolonged labour

D: Labour lasting more than 12 h after the onset of active labour.

A: Uterine dysfunction (hypotonic or infrequent contraction) from dehydration, acidosis, analgesia, antihypertensives; other underlying causes: abnormal pelvic shape/size; malpresentation (e.g. brow); malposition (e.g. occipitoposterior); excess pain/anxiety (release tocolytic adrenalin); cervical dystocia (from previous trauma/surgery); fetal macrosomia; obstruction by fibroids (rare); maternal exhaustion.

A/R: Primiparity ($\times$ 2) especially uterine hypotonia; cephalopelvic disproportion (? associated with past history of malposition); past history of pelvic fracture (abnormal pelvic shape); failure of head to engage antenatally; epidural analgesia.

E: 5–8 %.

H: Long labour: *First stage*: long latent phase (onset of contractions to cervical dilation, e.g. in primigravid with inefficient uterine contraction); cervical dilation < 0.5 cm/h (prolonged active phase e.g. in primigravid with inefficient uterine contraction); secondary arrest of cervical dilation (? obstruction). *Second stage*: > 3 h. ? associated backache (occipitoposterior position).

E: ? Maternal exhaustion; abdomen: ? scaphoid abdomen (occipitoposterior position), palpate for lie and presentation, palpate strength and frequency of contractions; internal examination: assess cervical dilation (normally 1 cm/h first stage) and descent of presenting part, position, ? pelvic size (for cephalopelvic disproportion).

P: n/a

I: *Bloods*: group and save (if surgery envisaged). *CTG*: fetal well-being/frequency, strength and duration of uterine contractions. *? Fetal scalp sampling*: if signs of fetal distress.

M: Treat past history of LSCS with caution (risk rupture) → trial of scar (e.g. 6 h). Treat any malposition/malpresentation accordingly.
Conservative: decrease maternal anxiety (and therefore adrenalin), e.g. partner support, environment.
Medical: amniotomy especially in delayed second stage; augmentation of labour with Syntocinon IV infused until three contractions/10 min—caution with past history of LSCS, exclude other causes of slow labour.
Instrumental delivery: ventouse preferred (less trauma/maternal analgesia required).
Surgical: CS; when instrumental delivery too difficult or unsuitable, cervical dystocia.

C: ↑ Intervention; ↑ maternal morbidity; maternal psychological trauma; ↑ fetal morbidity; fetal distress (also with Syntocinon); maternal exhaustion; maternal dehydration; maternal infection; ↑ post-partum haemorrhage; uterine rupture; vesicovaginal fistulae.

P: Dependent on underlying cause, monitoring and efficacy of interventions. Generally good.

Prolonged pregnancy

D: Pregnancy which proceeds beyond 42 weeks.

A: Undetermined in most cases.

A/R: Previous prolonged pregnancy, family history, oligohydramnios, fetal anencephaly.

E: 5 % pregnancies.

H: Continuation of pregnancy 2 weeks after EDD, ± decreased fetal movement. ? Accurately dated pregnancy (how was it calculated?, LMP, dating USS before/after 18 weeks' gestation).

E: Fundal height (twice a week), ? abnormal position, ? abnormal liquor volume.

P: No pathology/anencephaly.

I: Accurately date pregnancy (from history and previous investigation results), USS (liquor volume, fetal growth, developmental abnormality, placenta), CTG.

M: Sweep the membranes (↑ incidence of spontaneous labour > 40 weeks), induction of labour (↓ incidence of fetal distress, perinatal mortality), ? expectant management + ↑ fetal surveillance.

C: Uteroplacental insufficiency, intrapartum hypoxia, meconium aspiration syndrome, intrauterine death, slight ↑ birth injuries, perinatal morbidity (slight ↑ cerebral palsy, neonatal convulsions).

P: Perinatal mortality 9.7 in 1000, recurrence 30–40 % in subsequent pregnancies.

Puerperal psychosis

D: Puerperal psychiatric disorder involving hallucinations, delusions, disorder of affect and lack of insight.

A: ? Abrupt decrease of oestrogen, progesterone levels, ? increase in dopamine receptor sensitivity.

A/R: Family/personal history of affective disorder, previous history of psychosis. Single, primiparous. Instrumental delivery, CS, puerperal infection, perinatal death.

E: 1 in 1000 new mothers.

H: Abrupt onset 2–4 weeks after delivery. Majority present with depression, but 1/3 may present with mania (elevated/irritable mood, disinhibition, distractibility, overactivity, overspending, aggression, pressure of speech, flight of ideas, reduced sleep), hallucinations, delusions, confusion, lack of insight.

E: **Mother:** disinhibition, inappropriate dress,
Baby: evidence of neglect.

P: No identifiable pathology.

I: No investigation required.

M: Psychiatric evaluation (including suicide risk and risk to baby). Admission to psychiatric unit (specialist mother-and-baby unit if possible). Oral antidepressant drugs, neuroleptics (use with caution if breastfeeding). NB Evidence for use of oestrogen. ? ECT.

C: Suicide, neglect of child, inappropriate care, deliberate harm, infanticide.

P: Good short-term prognosis. 20% recurrent puerperal psychosis. 50% recurrent psychotic episode.

Puerperal pyrexia

D: A rise in maternal body temperature to 38°C in the first 24 h following delivery.

A: Endometritis (most common), UTI, perineal infection, wound infection, mastitis, respiratory tract infection. Endometritis caused by ascending bacteria (streptococcus, staphylococcus or *Escherichia coli*) from lower genital tract, UTI commonly caused by *E. coli*, wound, perineal and mastitis commonly caused by staphylococcus. DVT may cause mild, low-grade pyrexia and should be excluded.

A/R: Generalized ↑ risk: malnutrition, exhaustion, anaemia, underlying chronic disease.
Genital tract infection: prolonged labour/rupture of membranes, retained products of conception, multiple VEs, fetal blood sampling, operative delivery, episiotomy, perineal trauma.
UTI: post-partum perineal pain → incomplete bladder emptying, and catheterization.
Mastitis: breastfeeding.
Respiratory tract infection: immobility, especially if operative delivery.

E: 1–3 % of women following delivery.

H: Fever, malaise, SOB, lower abdominal pain, tenderness and/or purulent discharge from the source of the infection (e.g. purulent lochia), dysuria. An abscess may cause a swinging pyrexia.

E: General: septic shock (uncommon), pyrexia, tachycardia.
Respiratory: signs of consolidation.
Breast: tender, hard, erythematous, hot, purulent discharge (mastitis).
Abdomen: tender bulky uterus, wound infection.
Pelvic: perineal trauma, offensive bloodstained lochia.
Lower limb: evidence of DVT.

P: n/a

I: Infection screen: *Bloods*: FBC (↑ WCC), ESR, U&E, culture × 3, D-dimers (DVT). *Urine*: MSU. *Others*: CXR, sputum culture, HVS, wound swab, venogram (if suspected DVT).

M: Broad-spectrum antibiotics for 5 days to include cover for anaerobic organisms, e.g. metronidazole and amoxicillin. Antipyrexial drugs and analgesia if required. Perform ERPC if placental fragments on USS or no improvement within 24 h.

C: Septicaemia.

P: Low mortality and morbidity associated with thorough investigation and correct treatment. Deaths are more likely to be associated with delay in treatment and investigation.

Rhesus isoimmunization (RhI) and Rhesus disease (RhD)

D: RhI: development of antibodies within a Rhesus (Rh) negative individual, against one of the Rhesus antigens (C, D or E).
RhD: haemolytic anaemia in a Rh-positive fetus/neonate following the transfer of Rh antibodies from the mother.

A: RhI: 1- After receiving a transfusion incompletely cross-matched to Rh antigens.
2- Maternal exposure to fetal Rh antigens (large feto-maternal bleed, Rh-positive fetus).
RhD: transfer of Rh D antibody (most frequently) from mother to fetus → weakening of the envelopes of red blood cells and destruction within the spleen.

A/R: RhI: third stage labour, APH, spontaneous miscarriage, ectopic pregnancy, therapeutic abortion, amniocentesis, ECV.
RhD: previous maternal isoimmunization, small feto-maternal bleed (common).

E: Rh negativity most common in white people (15 %).
RhI: 1 % isoimmunization in first and 3–5 % in subsequent pregnancies (without prophylaxis).

H: Asymptomatic/↓ fetal movement. History of transfusion, previous jaundiced/hydrops baby, stillbirth, neonatal death.

E: RhI: no signs.
RhD: *Fetus*: polyhydramnios. *Neonate*: anaemia, jaundice, oedema, hydropic (oedema of skin, pleural effusion, ascites, hepatosplenomegaly).

P: RhD: antibody-mediated weakening of fetal red blood cell envelopes.

I: Screening (all women): *Bloods*:
1 *Booking*: Rh status + anti-D level (+ Rh status in partner if Rh-negative).
2 *28–36 weeks*: anti-D level (+ more frequently if anti-D detected).
3 *After birth* (cord blood): ABO and Rh group, Hb, direct Coombs, bilirubin.
At-risk fetus: *Bloods*: indirect Coombs; USS (hydrops fetalis), amniocentesis + spectrometry (AF bilirubin levels)/cordocentesis (blood group, haematocrit/Hb).

M: RhI: prevention: anti-D immunoglobulin given to all Rh-negative women at 28–34 weeks/within 72 h of likely feto-maternal bleed. After first trimester increase dose if Kleihauer test (detects level of fetal cells in maternal blood) is positive.
RhD: if rising anti-D levels detected/USS evidence anaemia/? fetal movements (also 10 weeks before occurrence of complications in previous pregnancy) refer to fetal medicine unit for amniocentesis/cordocentesis (repeated every 2 weeks). Treat according to severity:
1 *fetus*: intrauterine transfusion, elect time of delivery;
2 *neonate*: phototherapy, resuscitation, exchange transfusion, top up transfusion.

C: RhI: RhD in subsequent pregnancies.
RhD: hydrops fetalis, intrauterine death, neonatal death.

P: Depends on severity of RhD.

Sexual dysfunction

D: Difficulties with sexual intercourse which are usually psychosomatic in origin.

A: Psychological and/or physical origins.

A/R: Restrictive upbringing, inadequate sex education, sexual abuse, traumatic first sexual experience, high expectations, ↑ age, menopause, psychiatric conditions (alcoholism, depression, anxiety disorders, body image disturbance), physical illness, childbirth, relationship problems, performance anxiety, limited foreplay.

E: Difficult to assess. Affects 5% of subfertile couples.

H: Sexual response can be subdivided into four phases:
1 *Desire*.
2 *Arousal*: subdivided into excitement (↑ clitoris size, ↑ vaginal lubrication and engorgment of vagina and uterus in women and erection in men) and plateau phase (excitement completed).
3 *Orgasm*: contractions of vagina, cervix and pelvic floor in women, ejaculation in men.
4 *Resolution*: genital organs return to normal size, intense feeling of relaxation.
Common problems may affect any of these phases. *Women*: inhibited desire/arousal, failure to achieve orgasm or difficulties with penetration (vaginismus, dyspareunia, phobias). *Men*: inhibited desire, impotence, premature/retarded ejaculation.

E: Usually normal.
Women: *Pelvic inspection*: structural abnormalities, vaginal atrophy.
Speculum: pain and/or difficulty with insertion.
Men: *Inspection*: structural abnormalities.

P: n/a

I: Exclude any physical cause if indicated, e.g. diabetes, PID, multiple sclerosis, autonomic dysfunction.

M:
1 Identify precise area of difficulty and any precipitating, predisposing and perpetuating factors.
2 Exclude any physical and pharmacological factors and manage appropriately if present.
3 Identify any psychiatric problems.
4 Sexual intercourse therapy: (i) education, communication skills and permission giving; (ii) sensate focus behavioural therapy (e.g. 1 week of non-genital pleasuring followed by 1 week of genital pleasuring followed by 1 week of intercourse so that partners can learn how to satisfy each other).
5 Medical therapy if appropriate, e.g. Viagra for impotence.
6 Review to assess progress.

C: ↓ Frequency and duration of intercourse, relationship problems, psychiatric problems, e.g. depression, anxiety, alcoholism, subfertility.

P: 70% overall success rate with therapy described above.

Sheehan's syndrome

- **D:** Pituitary failure as a result of necrosis of the anterior lobe of the pituitary gland.
- **A:** Severe haemorrhage may cause thrombosis of the vessels supplying anterior pituitary lobe resulting in necrosis. Posterior pituitary is protected owing to its rich arterial supply.
- **A/R:** Severe haemorrhage, especially PPH.
- **E:** Rare. ↓ Incidence as a result of improved management of PPH.
- **H:** History of massive PPH. Complete failure of endocrine function of gland → failure of lactation (↓ prolactin), lethargy, cold intolerance, weight gain, constipation (↓ TSH), hypotension, infection (↓ ACTH), amenorrhoea, breast atrophy, subfertility, ↓ pubic hair (↓ FSH and LH). In addition there may be headache, visual loss and cranial nerve palsy. Severity may vary and mild cases may present later with amenorrhoea.
- **E:** *General:* signs of pituitary failure, e.g. regression of secondary sexual characteristics, loss of body hair, fine facial wrinkles, muscle wasting, pale puffy face.
- **P:** During pregnancy the pituitary gland ↑ in size and demands for blood supply, and is therefore more susceptible to necrosis in the event of a severe haemorrhage. The metabolic demand of the gland is highest just after delivery because of ↑ output of oxytocin and prolactin, ↑ its susceptibility to necrosis further. Ischaemia and infarction of the cells in the pituitary gland result in necrosis of the whole gland, although there may be an area of functioning tissue around the edge.
- **I:** *Bloods:* FBC (↓ Hb), U&E, TFT, FSH:LH ratio. *Others:* pituitary function tests (e.g. 9 a.m. serum cortisol), MRI of pituitary.
- **M:** Difficult condition to manage.
  Medical: ↓ ACTH: hydrocortisone 10 mg PO 3 × per day, ↓ TSH; l-thyroxine 100–150 μg PO 1 × per day, HRT.
- **C:** Premature menopause, osteoporosis, infertility, hypothyroidism (myxoedema coma, anaemia, etc.), ↓ cortisol (electrolyte disturbances, hypoglycaemia).
- **P:** Depends on severity of infarct.

Shoulder dystocia

D: Difficulty in delivering the fetal shoulders after delivery of the head.

A: The posterior shoulder enters the pelvic inlet while the anterior rests behind the symphysis pubis and fails to rotate. Alternatively, both shoulders may be impacted in the anteroposterior or transverse/oblique diameter.

A/R: LGA, maternal diabetes, ↑ maternal weight, postmaturity.

E: 0.25–1 % incidence.

H: Prolonged labour, slow crowning, difficulty delivering head, slow rotation of occiput to lateral position.

E: ? Maternal exhaustion. Pelvic examination: assess cervical dilation, state of membranes and presenting part. If shoulder dystocia suspected, determine whether anterior shoulder arrested above pelvic brim (to determine management). ? Moulding of shoulders. ? Turtle-necking.

P: n/a

I: n/a. Usually acute emergency necessitating immediate delivery.

M: **McRoberts position**: patient placed in lithotomy with hips hyperflexed and abducted. Episiotomy. Suprapubic pressure applied to dislodge the impacted anterior fetal shoulder from the symphysis with gentle downward traction on the head, to deliver anterior shoulder. If not delivered, rotation necessary before traction is repeated.
Surgical: cephalic replacement with CS (Zavanelli manoeuvre)—high success rate and good fetal outcome; however, should be last resort. Symphysiotomy associated with maternal complications.
Other: examine baby for neurological/skeletal damage. ? Assessment of fetal weight in subsequent pregnancies.

C: **Fetal**: asphyxia and neurological damage; death; brachial plexus injuries (commonly Erb's palsy, also T1 and C8 injuries, rarely T4 injuries); fractured clavicle.
Maternal: prolonged second stage may lead to excessive blood loss; vaginal and cervical lacerations. (PPH)

P: Brachial plexus injuries occur in 7–16 % of cases. Skeletal injuries occur in roughly 15 %.

C_5-C_6 → Erbs
C_7-T_1 - klumpkes

Thromboembolic disease

D: Condition in which a thrombus formed at one point in the circulation, becomes detached, is propelled by blood flow and lodges in a distal vessel.

A: Thrombus formation initiated by endothelial injury/stasis/hypercoagulability (Virchow's triad). Commonly occurs in deep veins of leg/pelvis and embolizes to pulmonary vasculature.

A/R: Obstetrics: pregnancy, CS (especially if emergency), instrumental delivery, prolonged labour, multiple pregnancy, high parity, pre-eclampsia, puerperium.
Gynaecology: oestrogen therapy, e.g. COC (increased risk if smoker); hyperemesis/dehydration; ovarian hyperstimulation syndrome; HRT; pelvic mass, gynaecological malignancy; pelvic surgery.
General: age, family/personal history, thrombophilia, obesity, varicose veins, infection, immobility, smoking, heart/lung disease.

E: Major direct cause of maternal death (UK).
PE: 1 in 6000 pregnancies, < 0.5 in 1000 COC users per year.

H: DVT: calf pain, leg swelling/lower abdominal pain, very rarely vaginal bleed (if iliofemoral).
PE: pleuritic chest pain, dyspnoea, cough, haemoptysis, history (PE/DVT).

E: DVT: unilateral leg oedema, calf tenderness, Homan's sign (calf tenderness on dorsiflexion of foot), tachycardia, low-grade pyrexia, palpable veins in vaginal fornices/lower abdomen (if iliofemoral thrombosis).
PE: tachypnoea, tachycardia, cyanosis, hypotension, gallop rhythm, ↑ JVP, coarse crackles, pleural rub sudden collapse.

P: DVT: venous thrombi usually in small veins (leg/pelvis).
PE: thrombus occlusion of pulmonary vessel.

I: DVT: Doppler ultrasound (tibial, femoral veins), venography.
PE: *Bloods*: FBC, ABG, plasma D-dimers, platelets (coagulation screen—only if difficulty in excluding amniotic fluid embolism, also for monitoring treatment). *Others*: ECG imaging, VQ scan (gold standard), CXR, pulmonary angiogram, spiral CT.

M: Prevention: risk assessment (before surgery/CS, OCP use, antenatal care), change contraception before surgery, early mobilization.
Low: compression stockings (during/after surgery or labour).
Moderate: Pre-/postoperative/post-delivery prophylactic heparin/LMW heparin.
High: higher dose heparin/LMW heparin.
Treatment: anticoagulation (DVT/PE): 5000 IU IV stat followed by 1000 IU/h IV infusion (check APTT after 6 h) *or* enoxaparin 1 mg/kg BD, then continue on warfarin PO/LMW heparin SC. Screen for thrombophilia after stopping treatment.
PE: cardiopulmonary resuscitation if collapsed, 60 % oxygen, ventilatory support (if needed), streptokinase 250 000 IU IV over 30 min, then 100 000 IU/h for 24 h, adequate analgesia, IV fluids/inotropes (if severe). Anticoagulate.

C: DVT: deep vein insufficiency, leg oedema, cramps, discoloration, ulceration, PE.
PE: shock, cardiovascular collapse, death.

P: Each year PE kills 15 women during pregnancy and in the puerperium in the UK, accounting for ∼1 in 3 direct maternal deaths.

Toxic shock syndrome

D: A syndrome of fever, erythematous rash, hypotension, diarrhoea and, in extreme cases, renal failure caused by *Staphylococcus aureus* endotoxin release into the bloodstream.

A: *S. aureus* produces toxic shock syndrome toxin (TSST:1) resulting in release of bradykinin, tumour necrosis factor and other biological response markers which cause systemic symptoms.

A/R: Tampons of higher absorbency, ↓ frequency of tampon change, overnight tampon use.

E: Rare in UK, < 1 in 25 000 tampon users.

H: Sudden onset of pyrexia > 39 °C, myalgia, rash, vomiting, diarrhoea, sore throat and headache. Usually presents on second to fourth day of menstruation.

E: **General:** shock (sepsis), oedematous and blanching erythematous rash resembling sunburn. Desquamation of palms and soles (1–2 weeks later). **Pelvic:** menstruating, tampon use.

P: *S. aureus* is a Gram-positive aerobic organism. Identified by microscopy (shows Gram-positive (purple) cocci arranged in clusters) and positive coagulase test. Culture on blood agar → creamy/white colonies.

I: *Bloods*: FBC (↑ WCC, ↓ plts), U&E, LFT (↑), serum BR (↑), creatine phosphokinase (↑) group and save, blood culture × 3. *Others*: HVS and culture of tampon.

M: Resuscitate shocked patients. Supportive therapy, e.g. dialysis for renal failure. IV flucloxacillin.

C: Septic shock, organ failure, DIC, ARDS, death.

P: Relapse can occur with subsequent menstruation, so advise against tampon use until *S. aureus* has been eradicated from genital tract.

84 Trichomonas vaginalis infection of female genital tract

D: Infection in the lower genital tract caused by presence of *Trichomonas vaginalis*.

A: An STI which is often asymptomatic in men.

A/R: Sexual contact

E: Currently uncommon sexually transmitted disease in UK.

H: Asymptomatic. Profuse, greenish/grey, frothy discharge which may have 'fishy' odour. Vaginal and vulval irritation. Dyspareunia.

E: Pelvic: *Inspection*: vaginal discharge, and vulval erythema. *Cusco speculum*: cervicitis. Erythematous, punctuate appearance of cervix (strawberry cervix).

P: *T. vaginalis* is a flagellate protozoa which shelters in the crypts of the vaginal epithelium and becomes a pathogen under conditions that raise the vaginal pH to 5.5.
Microscopy: motile flagellate protozoa seen. WBC often present.

I: Diagnostic: Vaginal pH > 5.0. HVS for direct microscopy and culture in a *Trichomonas* medium.
STI screen: HVS (BV, *Candida albicans*), endocervical swab (*Neisseria gonorrhoea*, *Chlamydia trachomatis*), blood tests for HIV, syphillis and hepatitis B.

M: Advice: contact tracing, contraception.
Medical: metronidazole (200 mg orally 3 × per day for 1 week or 2 g stat dose) or Flagyl (3 g orally stat dose). Repeat swab after 1 week. Follow-up examination after 2 months.

C: PID (ascending infection), premature delivery (if infected while pregnant), side-effects of treatment (flushing, headache, nausea, etc.).

P: 90 % cured with first course of metronidazole.

Umbilical cord prolapse

D: The presence of a loop of umbilical cord below the fetal presenting part following membrane rupture.

A: Segment of cord able to pass through cervical canal if the fetal presenting part is not closely applied to the lower uterine segment, or its engagement in the pelvis is interfered with.

A/R: Abnormal lie, malpresentation, cephalopelvic disproportion, placenta praevia (types 1 and 2), twin pregnancy, prematurity, amniotomy, version of the fetus.

E: 1 in 500 deliveries.

H: Membrane rupture with loop of cord seen or felt within or outside the vagina.

E: Palpable or visible cord in the vagina, cord pulsations may be felt.

P: n/a

I: *CTG*: deep variable decelerations or profound and prolonged decelerations. *Bloods*: FBC, group and save serum (results not usually ready before CS).

M: Displace presenting part manually: avoid handling cord (causes cord spasm). Fill bladder with 500–700 mL normal saline. Knee–chest position (kneeling with head down) until immediate CS. Forceps delivery/breech extraction (if cervix fully dilated + fetal head or breech engaged). Await delivery (if fetus dead and in longitudinal lie).

C: Fetal asphyxia, brain damage, death.

P: Good if prolapse occurs and is managed well in hospital. Morbidity and mortality increase with longer time to delivery interval but are more associated with prematurity and low birth weight (rather than birth asphyxia).

Urge incontinence

D: Also known as detrusor instability or overactivity. Spontaneous, uninhibited bladder contractions.

A: Often idiopathic. ? Results from bladder outlet obstruction. ? Sign of neurological disease.

A/R: Unknown, role of psychological factors not substantiated.

E: Second most common form of incontinence after USI in developed countries. Mainly postmenopausal women.

H: Urinary frequency, urgency, incontinence, nocturia, sometimes voiding difficulties. ? Symptoms of underlying neurological disorder.

E: Physical examination normal. Exclude vaginal prolapse, pelvic mass (including pregnancy) and neurological cause (neurological examination).

P: Involuntary contractions of the detrusor muscle occur spontaneously or with filling of the bladder.

I: MSU: exclude UTI/glycosuria (diabetes); ? cystoscopy (rule out bladder stones/tumours); urodynamics—filling cystometry—bladder filled via a catheter and detrusor pressure measured by subtracting abdominal pressure (measured via rectal pressure transducer) from intravesical pressure (measured via urethral transducer). ? Characteristically large detrusor pressure on filling with detrusor overactivity.

M: Medical: anticholinergics (e.g. propantheline, amitriptyline) especially-tolterodine (Detrusitol) and musculotropic relaxants (e.g. oxybutynin) (reduce frequency and urgency; however, limited by side-effects); desmopressin (? aid nocturia by decreasing urine volume); topical oestrogen therapy (? in some postmenopausal women).

Surgical: rarely used. Reserved for intractable cases (e.g. ileal conduit, clam cystoplasty).

Other: bladder retraining: regular voiding schedule, with progressively increasing time intervals to retrain the bladder to retain increasingly larger volumes; avoidance of diuretics e.g. alcohol, caffeine; fluid restriction (especially before bedtime); ? pelvic floor exercises—USI often coexists; reassurance; referral to an incontinence team; use of incontinence aids if appropriate.

C: Psychological sequelae of incontinence.

P: Symptoms may recur; however, remission can often be achieved again.

Urinary fistula

D: An abnormal communication between two epithelial-lined organs; in this case either ureter, bladder or urethra and the bowel, uterus, vagina or skin.

A: Pelvic malignancy, especially cervical carcinoma, radiotherapy, surgical trauma (CS), abdominal/vaginal hysterectomy, prolonged labour, diverticular disease.

A/R: As aetiology.

E: Uncommon. Most common cause in developed world: surgery and malignancy. And in developing world: prolonged labour.

H: **Ureterovaginal/vesicovaginal**: constant feeling of wetness/leakage. NB. History of difficult labour or malignancy.
Rectovaginal: ? faecal incontinence.

E: Direct inspection (use Sims' speculum). ? Fistula visualized—often difficult. ? Evidence of urine/faeces and excoriation of the skin.

P: **Most common types**: vesicovaginal, ureterovaginal.
Malignancy: associated with deep penetration.
Prolonged labour: avascular necrosis may occur from compression of the bladder base between the fetal head and pubic bone. Sloughing occurs after a few days followed by fistula formation.
Irradiation: vascular damage resulting in secondary ischaemic tissue damage.
Postoperative: damage from direct trauma or impaired blood supply from clamping, kinking, etc.

I: EUA and cystoscopy—visualization often difficult; cystogram and IVP—to illustrate site; MSU—exclude UTI. Fistulography may be required in difficult cases.

M: **Medical**: some small fistulae may heal spontaneously. Prolonged indwelling catheterization (? rests bladder). Antibiotics (prophylaxis).
Surgical: fistula repair—non-viable tissues surrounding fistula dissected out and fistula closed in layers. Vaginally for low fistulas and abdominally for higher ones (see bladder repair procedures, p. 99); ? ileal conduit/urinary diversion into the ileum if repair mot possible.
Other: reassurance. Advice from an incontinence team/use of incontinence aids explained if surgery is not possible/unsuccessful. Avoid vaginal delivery in subsequent pregnancies. Preventative measures important. Early diagnosis important for better prognosis.

C: Urinary infection, skin excoriation/infection, psychological sequelae of incontinence.

P: Variable depending on cause. 70 % success rate for non-malignant causes.

Urodynamic stress incontinence (previously genuine stress incontinence)

D: Involuntary loss of urine when intravesical pressure exceeds that of maximum urethral closure pressure in the absence of detrusor activity.

A: Mechanisms resulting in USI include:
1 failure of pelvic floor to support bladder neck and proximal urethra;
2 ↓ maximal closed urethral pressure (e.g. urethral stenosis/scarring).
Factors contributing to these include:
1 *Congenital*: epispadias, collagen defects;
2 *Pelvic floor damage*: childbirth, pelvic surgery;
3 *Urethral damage*: radiotherapy, recurrent UTI, urethral surgery;
4 *Chronic ↑ intra-abdominal pressure*: chronic cough, constipation, pelvic mass;
5 *Menopause*.

A/R: Prolonged active second stage labour, baby > 4 kg, instrumental delivery, multiparity, obesity, ↑ age.

E: > 10 % women affected following childbirth. > 50 % cases of incontinence are caused by USI.

H: Stress incontinence (urine loss when laughing, coughing, etc.), urge incontinence (urine loss with sudden desire to void), frequency (voiding > 6 × per day), urgency (sudden desire to void), feeling of 'something coming down' if associated with prolapse.

E: (with Sims' speculum): prolapse, incontinence when patient coughs.

P: **Congenital:** epispadias—failure of midline fusion of mesoderm, resulting in widened bladder neck, separation of pubic symphysis and shortened urethra. Defective collagen structure if disorder of collagen synthesis, e.g. Ehlers–Danlos syndrome, osteogenesis imperfecta.
Acquired: unknown. ? Pudendal nerve damage and/or ischaemic damage during second stage of labour.

I: MSU (UTI), Dipstix (glycosuria, haematuria), urinary diary, pad test (1 h), cystometry (to determine loss of urine with no increase in detrusor pressure), urethral pressure profile, uroflowmetry, postvoiding USS/catheterization.

M: **Conservative:** use if patient refuses or unfit for surgery, mild symptoms, accompanying detrusor overactivity, family incomplete. Options include:
1 pelvic floor exercises (± perineometry);
2 vaginal cones;
3 maximal electrical stimulation;
4 vaginal devices (Contigard, sponge tampons, Intro bladder neck prothesis);
5 urethral devices (Reliance Insert);
6 pharmacological (α-adrenergic agonists).
Surgery: most effective way of curing patient. Aim is to elevate the bladder neck. Procedure employed depends on patient (for details on procedures employed see p. 99). Options include:
1 Burch colposuspension;
2 tension-free vaginal tape;
3 anterior repair procedure via vagina;
4 macroplastique;
5 Raz/Pererya/Stamey procedure.
Options 1–3 are the most frequently used.

Urodynamic stress incontinence (previously genuine stress incontinence) continued

P: 40–60 % show improvement with conservative treatment if symptoms mild. Most patients with more severe symptoms will require surgery (~90 % success rate). Effects of Stamey or Raz procedure last for approximately 2 years.

C: **Psychosocial:** social embarrassment, sexual dysfunction.
Complications of surgery: urinary retention, DI, urethral damage, etc.

Uterine inversion

D: Inversion of the fundus either into the uterine cavity, through the cervix or even outside the vagina following delivery.

A: Majority are iatrogenic, secondary to strong force applied to umbilical cord that is attached to a placenta located in the fundus and has not yet separated.

A/R: Tough cord, ↑ adherence of placenta (e.g. placenta accreta), fundal implantation of placenta, multiparity (lax uterine muscles), sudden bearing down effort.

E: Rare.

H: Haemorrhage (90 %), pain, shock (40 %)—may be out of proportion to blood loss because of ↑ vagal tone.

E: General: shock (↓ BP, tachycardic, pale, clammy, etc.).
Abdomen: cannot feel uterine fundus.
Pelvic: in second or third degree cases uterine fundus will be seen in or outside the vagina. A first degree case is diagnosed by feeling the fundus at the top of the vagina.

P: Classified as:
1 *First degree*: inverted at the external os;
2 *Second degree*: fundus protrudes into vagina;
3 *Third degree*: uterus, cervix and vagina prolapse outside the vulva.

I: *Bloods*: FBC (↓ Hb), cross-match 6 units.

M: An emergency that can be fatal if not treated correctly.
Immediate:
1 Summon senior help.
2 Attempt manual reduction without attempting to remove the placenta by applying an upwards pressure along the long axis of the vagina to the fundus, with the palm of the hand.
3 If unsuccessful, gain IV access (two large-bore cannulae) and administer colloid. Anaesthetize and give tocolytic drugs IV, e.g. ritodrine, to promote uterine relaxation and aid reduction.
4 A further attempt is made at manual reduction under GA by applying pressure to the part that was last to invert. If successful, tocolytics stopped and ergometrine IV given while performing bimanual compression until a firm uterine contraction is achieved. If unsuccessful, perform O'Sullivan's hydrostatic method (step 5).
5 Uterus is held in vagina and the introitus sealed by the attendant's hands. 2 L warm saline is quickly infused into the vagina, causing the walls to distend and fundus to rise until the inversion is corrected. Give ergometrine IV and perform bimanual compression until a contraction is achieved.
6 If this fails, perform laparotomy for reduction via abdominal route.
Following reposition: examine genitourinary tract for trauma. Monitor renal function. Observe for signs of sepsis.

C: Death, post-partum infection, renal failure, strangulation and necrosis of uterus, subacute/chronic inversion if undiagnosed.

P: Most cases can be managed without surgical intervention. 30 % cases can be reduced immediately.

Uterine rupture

- **D:** Development of a tear in the uterine wall.
- **A:** Rupture of weak surgical scar in late pregnancy or labour; spontaneous rupture in labour; trauma.
- **A/R:** Scar rupture (previous CS—especially classical (higher) incision, myomectomy/other uterine surgery); spontaneous rupture (obstructed labour, use of oxytocic agents, multiparity, congenital uterine abnormality); trauma (high forceps delivery, breech extraction, perforating trauma), extension of a cervical tear.
- **E:** Rare, 1 in 1500 deliveries.
- **H:** Vaginal bleeding, constant lower abdominal pain (mild/severe), cessation of contractions. ? Later shock.
- **E:** Fetal distress. Vaginal bleeding: APH/PPH. Maternal tachycardia/sudden shock: tachycardia, hypotension, pallor, cold sweaty peripheries. Absent fetal heart sounds, cessation of contractions, recession of presenting part.
- **P:** **Complete/incomplete:** tear through uterine wall and serosal peritoneal coat/tear in uterine wall not involving peritoneal coat. Although of little practical importance in obstetrics.
  Spontaneous rupture: lower uterine segment often thin and overstretched.
  Scar rupture: weak scar (imperfect healing, inaccurate suturing of edges, implanted placenta, repeat CS through old scar).
- **I:** *Bloods*: FBC, clotting factors, cross match 6 units, may require type-specific blood. *CTG*: fetal distress? *Imaging*: abdominal USS may be helpful to aid diagnosis/excluded differential diagnosis in early cases.
- **M:** IV access (two large-bore cannulae)—replace fluids. Urgent laparotomy, deliver baby, repair/remove uterus. Provide antibiotic cover, pain relief. NB Need informed consent; explain ↑ probability hysterectomy/subtotal hysterectomy.
- **C:** **Mother:** haemorrhage, shock, infection, bladder/urethral injury, DIC, infertility/sterility, death.
  Fetus: fetal/neonatal death, neonatal morbidity.
- **P:** Maternal mortality 5 %; fetal mortality 30 %.

Uterovaginal prolapse

D: Protrusion of vagina and/or uterus outside of its normal anatomical boundaries. Types include: uterine (Ut), cystocele (C), urethrocele (Ur), rectocele (R) and enterocele (E).

A: Unknown.

A/R: Levator ani muscle forms floor of pelvis and supports vaginal walls. Vaginal walls and cardinal ligaments (extend from pelvic wall → cervix). Denervation and ischaemic damage result in weakness of these supports. Predisposing and precipitating factors include **PROLAPSE**:
Pregnancy (multiparity, baby > 4.0 kg)
Race (↑ white women)
Oestrogen deficiency
Labour (prolonged 2nd stage, pushing before fully dilated, intervention
Anatomy (short vagina)
Pelvic surgery
Strain on supports (chronic cough, constipation, obesity, lifting heavy weights)
Elastin and collagen abnormalities (e.g. Ehlers–Danlos).

E: Common, ~20 % of women following childbirth.

H: Asymptomatic, dragging/lump in vagina (worse on standing/at end of day). **Specific:** *Ut*: urinary symptoms (stress incontinence, frequency, recurrent UTI), lower backache, bloodstained discharge (with procidentia). *C and U*: urinary symptoms. *R*: constipation, difficulty passing stool (may require manual reduction prior to bowel movement), lower backache.

E: Pelvic: *Inspection*: procidentia. *Bimanual*: lax vaginal walls, bulge, cervix low down in vagina. *Sims' speculum in left lateralor 3/4 prone position*: prolapse, stress incontinence when bears down. *PR* (to distinguish between rectocele and enterocele): finger in rectum will bulge into rectocele, but not enterocele.

P: Prolapse classified according to degree and anatomical site.
Degree: *First degree*: descent within vagina. *Second degree*: descent to introitus. *Third degree*: extends beyond introitus. *No evidence → all thru in vce*
Anatomical site: *Ut*: always occurs with vaginal prolapse. In severe cases cervical epithelium may become keratinized. *C*: anterior wall prolapse containing bladder. *Ur*: lower anterior wall prolapse containing urethra. *R*: posterior wall containing rectum. *E*: prolapse of pouch of Douglas, usually contains small bowel.

I: Diagnostic: Pelvic USS, endometrial biopsy if PMB, MSU and urodynamics if urinary symptoms, rectal physiology studies if defaecation problems.
Fitness for surgery: FBC, U&E, group and save, CXR and ECG if necessary.

M: Advice: lifestyle (↓ weight, stop smoking, avoid heavy physical work).
Conservative (for relief of symptoms while awaiting surgery, unfit for surgery or childbearing not complete): physiotherapy, ring/shelf pessaries. *c̄ topical cream*
Surgical: *C*: uterovesical suspension, TVT. *Ut*: hysterectomy/Manchester repair. *E*: uterosacral suspension. *R*: posterior colporrhaphy. *Total Vault prolap → sac*
Prevention: better management of labour and trauma brought about by delivery, pelvic floor exercises, HRT.

C: *C*: ureteric obstruction. *E*: strangulation of small bowel. *Ut*: ulceration of cervix. *Surgery*: urinary retention, infection, incontinence, sexual dysfunction.

P: Most cases require surgery to ease symptoms, which is successful in majority of patients.

Vaginismus

- **D:** Spasm of the pelvic floor muscles resulting in difficult or painful penetration into the vagina.
- **A:** Unknown, strong psychological component.
- **A/R:** Phobia; anxiety; past history of sexual abuse.
- **E:** <2% of women.
- **H:** Dyspareunia; inability to have penetrative intercourse; difficulty with tampon use.
- **E:** Some patients may not be able to tolerate pelvic examination.
- **P:** n/a
- **I:** Exclude vaginal infection (e.g. *Candida albicans*, *Trichomonas vaginalis*, etc.)/other causes of dyspareunia.
- **M:** Vaginal dilators of gradually increasing sizes placed in vagina by patients (aid muscle relaxation). Pelvic floor excercises. Relaxation techniques. 'Guided tour' (familiarization with external genitalia). Psychological intervention/behavioural therapy.
- **C:** Psychological sequelae; inability to conceive; relationship issues.
- **P:** Protracted treatment. Progression to penile penetration may be difficult.

Vulval intraepithelial neoplasia

D: Presence of atypical cells within vulval epithelium. Vulval equivalent of CIN.

A: Unknown. ? Human papilloma virus types 16, 18 and 31.

A/R: CIN (30 % of VIN cases also have CIN), lichen sclerosus, squamous hyperplasia of the vulva, recurrent infection, immunosuppression (e.g. transplant patients), granulomatous disease, smoking.

E: Increasing but less common than CIN. Affects all age groups. 40 % <40 years.

H: 20 % asymptomatic. Pruritus vulvae, pain.

E: Pelvic: lesions visible to naked eye. May be multifocal (more common in women <40 years) or unifocal. Can affect any part of the vulva (especially perineal skin, area around the clitoris and labia minora) Raised, rough, wart-like appearance, vary in size and colour (white, red or dark brown).

Application of 5 % acetic acid: VIN turns white with mosaic/punctate appearance.

P: Macro: white lesions resulting from hyperkeratinization, red lesions caused by thinning of the vulval epithelium and dark brown lesions caused by ↑ melanin deposition.
Micro: categories for VIN are the same as those used for CIN:
VIN I: atypical cells present in lower one-third of epithelium.
VIN II: atypical cells present in lower two-thirds epithelium.
VIN III: atypical cells present throughout the whole thickness of the epithelium (previously known as Bowen's disease).
Atypical cells: hyperchromatic, poorly defined, ↑ mitoses, multinucleated, ↑ nuclear : cytoplasmic ratio, ↑ cellular density.

I: Colposcopy of vagina and cervix (exclude CIN), biopsy of lesion (diagnostic).

M: Conservative: <45 years, asymptomatic, mild symptoms. Symptomatic relief with topical steroids. Observe for malignant change. Repeat biopsy if any suspicious changes.
Surgery: >45 years, moderate/severe symptoms, immunosuppressed. Consider laser therapy or skinning vulvectomy.

C: Malignant change, complications from surgery (discomfort, poor cosmetic results), recurrence.

P: Natural course of disease currently unknown. Recent research estimates 87 % of VIN III progress to invasive disease if not treated.

PROCEDURES

Amniocentesis

D: Sampling of amniotic fluid for prenatal diagnosis or therapy (amniodrainage).

I: **Diagnostic:** ↑ risk of chromosomal disorders (↑ age; family history; abnormal triple/double marker test); Rhesus/other blood group isoimmunization, ? congenital toxoplasmosis; estimation of fetal lung maturity (rare); neural tube defects (very rare).
Therapeutic: polyhydramnios.

M: Commonly at 16 weeks' gestation. Pre-procedure counselling. Using sterile technique, spinal needle inserted via maternal abdomen under ultrasound guidance into a pool of liquor avoiding the fetus/placenta. 10–20 mL amniotic fluid aspirated for diagnostic purposes/further amounts for drainage (polyhydramnios). Anti-D administered to Rhesus-negative mothers. Fluid-containing amniocytes and fetal cells cultured. ? Karyotyping; measurement OD450 (Rhesus isoimmunization); PCR (congenital toxoplasmosis); chromosomal analysis results take ~ 3–4 weeks. A quicker test is FISH. Results are available within 48 h.

A: Reliable method prenatal diagnosis.
Method of relieving maternal discomfort/preventing preterm labour with severe and acute polyhydramnios.
Least procedure-related loss for invasive prenatal diagnosis.
Allows termination before 22 weeks if appropriate.

D: 1 % attributable risk pregnancy loss at 16 weeks. 0.1 % risk obtaining wrong karyotype (maternal cells). As Complications.

C: Miscarriage.
? Low birthweight.
? Effects on pulmonary development (hypoplasia).
Rhesus isoimmunization.
Fetal trauma.
Chorioamnionitis.
Oligohydramnios and associated disorders (e.g. talipes).
PROM.
Arthrogryposis.

P: 1 % risk of pregnancy loss; however, other complications are less common.

Biophysical profile

D: An ultrasonographical assessment of fetal behaviour evaluating indicators of acute and chronic fetal hypoxia and placental function.

I: IUGR.
↓ Decreased fetal movement.
Maternal complications/past history of maternal complications.
Prolonged pregnancy.
Bleeding in pregnancy.
Abnormalities of amniotic fluid volume.
Suspicion of fetal compromise.

M: Ultrasound assessment (see Table P.1).

A: Combined parameters improve predictive value of individual measurements.
Non-invasive.
Can indicate the necessity for early delivery.

D: 10 % margin of error. Therefore twice weekly serial readings required.
Criteria assessed do not have equal importance.
Time consuming (~90 min)—more important parameters (e.g. heart rate) can be evaluated using quicker methods.

C: n/a

P: If no fetal growth abnormalities, IUD unlikely to occur within the next 2 weeks.

Table P.1 Ultrasound assessment.

	Normal	Abnormal
• Fetal tone	Flexion at rest, >1 episode extension of extremities/spine/hand and return to flexion	Extension at rest and no/partial return to flexion with movement
• Fetal body movements	>2 episodes of limb/trunk movement within 30 min	<2 episodes in 30 min
• Fetal breathing movements	1 or more episodes of ≥20 s within 30 min	Absent/short gasps <20 s within 30 min
• Amniotic fluid volume	1 or more pockets of fluid measuring ≥2 cm in vertical axis	Either no pockets or largest pocket <2 cm in vertical axis
• Fetal heart rate patterns	Reactive: 2 or more accelerations of ≥15 bmp for >15 s associated with fetal movement within 20 min	Non-reactive: <2 accelerations ≥15 bmp for >15 s within 20 min

Score given if these factors present. Normal score 2, abnormal score 0. Total scores of 8–10 are reassuring. Low score indicates possible fetal compromise.

Bladder suspension procedures for urodynamic stress incontinence

D: Surgical elevation of the bladder neck to alleviate symptoms of urodynamic stress incontinence (USI, see p. 88), previously known as genuine stress incontinence.

I: Confirmed USI and after conservative methods have failed, e.g. pelvic floor exercises, weight loss.

M: Retropubic procedures:
1 *Burch colposuspension*: appropriate for a cystocele accompanied by stress incontinence secondary to sphincter damage. The retropubic space is opened via a Pfannenstiel incision. The bladder neck is identified and suspended from the iliopectineal ligaments. This has a 90% success rate, but 10% develop *de novo* detrusor instability and 15% develop an enterocoele or rectocoele.
2 *Tension-free vaginal tape*: a more recent procedure where prolene tape is placed transvaginally supporting the urethra without adding tension. The ends of the tape are brought through a suprapubic incision. This method is thought to have much reduced associated morbidity.
3 *Marshall–Marchetti–Krantz procedure*: the bladder neck is supported from the periosteum of the symphysis pubis. Success rates and complications as for the Burch colposuspension, plus osteitis of pubic bone.
4 *Anterior colporrhaphy*: a vertical anterior wall incision is made to reveal part of the urethra, the urethrovesical junction and the bladder base. The urethrovesical junction is sutured to a higher level. The cystocoele is then reduced and sutured in place. The anterior wall is then sutured following removal of any excess tissue. Disadvantages include postoperative urinary retention and urethral sphincter damage resulting in incontinence. Less commonly used now.

Non-invasive: *Macroplastique*: injection of microparticulate silicone either periurethrally or transurethrally on either side of the bladder neck to 'bulk' it. <50% cure rate at 2 years, but 70% have an improvement in symptoms.

Sling procedures: two strips of fascia are sutured under the bladder neck and on to the abdominal rectus fascia. High success rate, but also has high rate of infection and postoperative urinary retention. Usually reserved for refractory incontinence with prolapse.

Transvaginal procedures: urethropexy is indicated for large anterior wall prolapse. Has a lower success rate than retropubic procedures and is used when more extensive procedures are medically contraindicated.

Laparoscopic procedures: the bladder neck is elevated by suturing the upper lateral vaginal walls to the iliopectineal ligaments under laparoscopic guidance.

A: Depends on methods used.

D: Common problems include UTI, urinary retention and incontinence as a result of sphincter damage.

P: Depends on cause and procedure used.

Caesarean section

D: Surgical delivery of viable fetus via abdomen. Performed in 20 % deliveries in UK.

I: When risk of vaginal delivery > risk of CS.
Elective: *Maternal*: placenta praevia, pre-eclampsia, severe PIH, pelvic abnormality, two or more previous CS, failed induction of labour, maternal illness (severe cardiac disease, diabetes), infection (HIV, active herpes simplex virus), older nulliparous women, maternal request. *Fetal*: malpresentation (breech, transverse, brow, face), multiple pregnancy, macrosomia, prematurity (< 34 weeks), severe IUGR.
Emergency: *Maternal*: failure to progress in labour (cephalopelvic disproportion, inefficient uterine action), placental abruption, cord prolapse, maternal distress. *Fetal*: fetal distress, malposition (occipitoposterior, occipitotransverse).

M: Patient anaesthetized (epidural or spinal block, GA used occasionally if patient requests or haemorrhage expected, e.g. placenta praevia) and catheterized. Table tilted 15° to left. Alternatively, mother may be tilted on to her left side.
Lower segment: performed in > 90 % because of lower rate of postnatal morbidity and improved cosmetic appearance. Transverse incision is made through lower uterine segment, after ensuring bladder is out of the way. Fetal presenting part is then delivered through incision with assistance of firm fundal pressure. Placenta is then delivered and uterine wound sutured in two layers.
Classical: may be used in prematurity (< 34 weeks) because of poorly formed lower uterine segment, placenta praevia, transverse lie with back facing down, cervical carcinoma and extensive adhesion preventing lower uterine segment from being reached. *De Lees* method (involves a shorter longitudinal incision) is used in extreme prematurity (< 28 weeks). Uterine wound is sutured in three layers to reduce incidence of dehiscence during uterine involution.
Following operation, advise early mobilization and to minimize physical work and driving for 6 weeks.

A: Relatively safe operation. ↓ Fetal morbidity. Preservation of pelvic floor muscles resulting in decreased incidence of GSI and urogenital prolapse is not proven as pelvic floor changes occur secondary to pregnancy alone, regardless of method of delivery.

D: Psychological: mother may feel as if she has 'failed' in some way.

C: Immediate: haemorrhage, damage to bladder, cervix or vagina.
Intermediate: infection (15 %) (uterine, wound, UTI)—prophylactic antibiotics are given to all women, urinary retention, TED—prophylactic subcutaneous heparin (LMW/fractionated heparin) is given to women at high risk (> 35 year, obese, anaemia, past history of TED), paralytic ileus, wound dehiscence (especially with a longitudinal incision).
Late: increased risk of uterine rupture with subsequent pregnancies (1 % with lower segment, 6 % with classical CS).
Neonate: increased incidence of respiratory distress syndrome, especially if premature, because of lack of normal stimulation to breathe.

P: Two-thirds will have vaginal delivery with next pregnancy if reason for CS is not recurring (e.g. pelvic abnormality).

Cardiotocograph

D: Electronic recording of FHR patterns and uterine activity

I: **Antenatally:** ↓ fetal movements, part of biophysical profile to assess fetal well-being.
Intrapartum: routine, 2–hourly, 15 min recording or after administration of prostaglandin gel/suppository. Continuous CTG if high-risk pregnancy (e.g. diabetes, poly-/oligohydramnios, maternal cardiac disease, evidence of uteroplacental insufficiency), IUGR, meconium, Syntocinon, epidural, previous CS, abnormal CTG. No evidence for value of continuous CTG in low-risk pregnancies.

M: Recording made using Doppler USS. Two transducers attached to mother's abdomen. One is placed at fundus of uterus to measure uterine activity. The other is placed to get optimal measurement of FH—usually over anterior shoulder of fetus. A fetal scalp electrode may also be used to measure FH if abdominal measurement fails to detect it or in the case of multiple pregnancies to measure FH of presenting fetus. The following variables are assessed.

1 *Baseline* (110–160 bpm): baseline bradycardia in maturity, sedation, fetal congenital heart disease. Baseline tachycardia in prematurity, fetal distress and maternal tachycardia (e.g. maternal pyrexia).
2 *Variability* (10–25 bpm): ? loss caused by fetal activity (sleep, sedation secondary to opiate analgesia), prematurity, fetal distress (especially if late decelerations also present).
3 *Accelerations* (≥ 2 of 15 bpm, lasting for 15 s over 15–min period = reactive trace): loss of reactivity caused by ↓ fetal activity and fetal distress.
4 *Decelerations* (15 bpm lasting for 15 s). *Early*: occur with contractions—physiological as a result of pressure on fetal head raising ICP and stimulating vagal tone. *Late* (> 15 s after contraction): serious, indicate fetal distress. *Variable*: cord compression or fetal distress (less common).

A: Assesses need for immediate delivery antenatally. *During labour*: highly sensitive for detecting fetal distress, ↓ short-term neurological complications, provides visual reassurance to parents.

D: FH is last to be affected by fetal compromise, therefore limited use in antenatal screening. Requires accurate interpretation. False reassurance results in ↑ perinatal mortality. Needs to be performed daily in high-risk pregnancies.
During labour: not specific (i.e. many normal babies are born who have had an abnormal CTG), restricts movement of mother, ↑ intervention, no proven ↓ in neonatal mortality, use of CTG alone ↑ CS rate (although this is offset with use of fetal blood sampling).

P: Currently unsuitable for screening at present, but with CT interpretation of variability it may be able to predict more accurately the risk of impending complications.

Cervical smear

D: Technique involving the collection and cytological examination of cervical cells.

I: **Cervical screening:** all sexually active women between 20 and 65 years.
First smear: 20 years/first year of sexual activity (if earlier).
Subsequent smears: 3–yearly intervals.
Follow-up: after colposcopy/cervical cancer treatment.

M: Explain procedure to patient.
Insert warmed speculum into vagina to expose cervix.
Take 360° scraping from squamocolumnar transformation zone using an Aylesbury/Ayres spatula or a cytobrush (endocervical sample).
Smear specimen over slide and add fixative immediately.
Send smear for cytological examination (presence/severity of dyskaryosis— mild, moderate or severe).
NB Also liquid-based cytology (avoids cell retention on spatula, avoids air drying).

A: Cervical screening programme:
Detects 91 % of premalignant changes (CIN);
Allows earlier treatment (more successful);
↓ Cervical cancer mortality rate.

D: False-negative results: error in smear taking, misinterpretation of results, clerical error.
False-positive results: misinterpretation, infection, pregnancy, clerical error.
Screening: does not reach all at-risk population.
Adequacy of sample may depend on site of transformation zone.

C: Cervical trauma.
Infection.

P: n/a.

Chorionic villous sampling

D: Biopsy of trophoblast by insertion of either a plastic or metal cannula through the cervix or by a needle through the abdomen.

I: Increased risk of fetal abnormality (chromosomal and autosomal dominant/recessive), e.g. abnormality detected (↑ nuchal fold thickness), older mothers, previous history of chromosomal abnormality or sex-linked disease. Chorionic tissue can also be examined for organisms, e.g. CMV or toxoplasma.

M: Transabdominal (TA) or transcervical (TC) approach can be used. TA route has ↓ risk of infection, ruptured membranes and abortion. TC approach may be more suitable for women with a low-lying posterior placenta or thick abdominal wall.

TA:
1 USS is used to determine position of placenta.
2 Local anaesthetic is infused to anaesthetize area.
3 CVS needle attached to syringe is inserted into placenta under USS guidance.
4 Small sample of tissue is removed and sent for analysis.

TC:
1 A catheter is inserted via a speculum through the cervix to the edge of placenta under USS guidance.
2 Small sample of tissue is removed and sent for analysis and immediate confirmation that villi have been obtained.

Analysis: *Direct preparation*: cytotrophoblast cells are examined directly to identify those in metaphase. Gives rapid results (< 48 h), but is subject to misinterpretation if 'confined placental mosaicism' is present (i.e. karyotype of placenta is different to that of fetus) so culture must also be carried out.

Culture: fibroblasts from villi core are examined. Results available after 10 days.

A: Performed earlier in pregnancy (11–14 weeks) than amniocentesis, allowing earlier TOP if requested. Rapid provisional results ↓ parental anxiety.

D: Karyotyping slightly less accurate than amniocentesis; ↑ risk of miscarriage.

C: Limb and facial deformities (especially of fingers and nose) if < 10 weeks. Risk of spontaneous abortion 1 % > background risk (~ 3–4 %).

P: n/a

Colposcopy

D: The use of a low-powered binocular (magnifies by 4–25 ×) microscope used in the examination of the transformation zone of the cervix.

I: Dyskaryosis detected at cervical smear. Criteria under guidance of British Society of Colposcopy and Cervical Pathology (BSCCP) recommend referral if moderate or severe dyskariosis or mild/borderline dykaryosis on two consecutive occasions 6 months apart. Women with cervical ectopy/eversion are also referred for colposcopy as the inflammatory process can mask underlying CIN on a cervical smear.

M:
1 The patient is placed in the lithotomy position and the cervix visualized using a bivalve speculum.
2 The colposcope is focused onto the cervix to identify areas of abnormality.
3 3–5% acetic acid is applied. This coagulates protein in the cytoplasm and nuclei of cells. Abnormal cells have an ↑ nucleoprotein density compared to normal cells. On application of acetic acid the cells become opaque, blocking out the colour from the underlying vasculature, and are seen as white to the naked eye. Colposcopy also allows the subepithelial vascular pattern and vaginal epithelium to be examined. Normal vaginal squamous epithelium is smooth and pale and the normal columnar epithelium of the cervical os is folded. Abnormal epithelium typically has either a mosaic vasculature, punctate pattern (suggestive of carcinoma in situ) or branching pattern (suggestive of invasive cancer).
4 Specific areas for biopsy are identified and samples taken if CIN suspected. Treatment may be given at this time (see CIN management).
5 Advice: abstain from intercourse and tampon use for 24 h if biopsy performed or for 2–3 weeks if treatment given.

A: Rapid, no anaesthesia required so can be performed on outpatient basis. Low risk of complications.

D: Unpleasant procedure. Risk of infection and bleeding. Always requires follow-up. ? Overtreatment and unnecessary colposcopy of low-grade premalignant change as ~50% of CIN I will spontaneously regress.

C: Infection, cervical trauma.

P: Bloodstained discharge is normal following biopsy or treatment.

Epidural

D: Local anaesthesia and opiate are injected via a catheter into the epidural space to alleviate pain by blocking the spinal nerves from the uterus and vagina (T10–L1). Blocks sensory (except pressure) and partially blocks motor nerones.

I: Pain relief during labour, anaesthesia for operative delivery. Medical indications include:
1 to ↓ BP in hypertensive women;
2 ↓ premature desire to push, e.g. premature delivery.

M: Carried out by skilled anaesthetist. Usually started in first stage of labour.
1 Patient is asked to bend forward while sitting on edge of bed to flex spine. Tuohy needle is then inserted into the space between L2 and L3.
2 Bupivacaine (usually used as longer duration of action compared to lignocaine (lidocaine)) is then infused through needle. Increasingly, a lower dose of bupivacaine is being used in combination with an opioid (fentanyl or pethidine) to reduce the motor blockade, allowing the patient to remain mobile ('mobile' epidural).
3 Polythene catheter is then threaded through the needle and left in place for 'top ups' at intervals. IV saline infusion is started to minimize the risk of hypotension as a result of vasodilation.
4 Maternal BP and HR are monitored at 5–min intervals for 20 min following a top up. A CTG is also performed.
5 Rapid anaesthesia for CS can be achieved by infusing a higher dose of lignocaine (lidocaine) (effect is quicker than bupivacaine) with a low dose of adrenaline (↓ absorption, therefore ↑ rate of effect). Epidural fentanyl (opioid) is also infused to ↓ risk of patient feeling pain during operation.

A: Rapid relief of pain in 95 % women. May speed up delivery by relaxing the pelvic muscles. Few long-term side-effects. Use in CS allows mother to see her baby immediately, and helps bonding. 'Low-dose' epidurals enable mother to remain mobile.

D: Requires ↑ medical supervision and monitoring. ↓ Desire to push in the second stage may ↑ the chances of instrumental delivery unless second stage managed differently, i.e. allow 2 h for passive stage instead of usual 1 h.

C: **Immediate complications:** total spinal shock, headache (caused by post-dural puncture or 'spinal tap'), dizziness, shivering, failure to establish block, epidural haematoma, transient fetal bradycardias, urinary retention because of ↓ bladder sensation, hypotension because of vasodilation or temporary respiratory muscle paralysis caused by accidental intrathecal infusion.
Delayed complications: weakness or parasthesia of the lower limbs (rare). Caution in pre-eclampsia because of ↑ risk of DIC, thus increased risk of bleeding.
Contraindicated in local sepsis, active neurological disease, hypovolaemia, anticoagulant therapy, bleeding diathesis and some cardiac diseases.

P: Most women have no significant side-effects and find labour more manageable.

Episiotomy

D: A deliberate incision into the perineum to enlarge the vaginal introitus with the aim of assisting the delivery of a fetus.

I: **Absolute:** previous perineal reconstructive surgery or pelvic floor surgery. **Relative:** if a tear as a result of a large baby or small introitus is otherwise inevitable, fetal hypoxia demanding a quick delivery, breech presentation, instrumental delivery, shoulder dystocia.

M: Inform patient of procedure.
1 Ensure perineum is distended and stretched by the fetal presenting part.
2 Unless epidural in site the perineum should be infiltrated with local anaesthetic.
3 Fetus protected with one hand while the other makes a clean incision into the perineum with large, sharp and straight scissors. Median incisions may suffice if only a small enlargement is required. This has the benefit of avoiding major arteries, easier to repair and ↓ pain and dyspareunia following delivery but ↑ chance of a tear into the rectal mucosa or anal sphincter. J-shaped or mediolateral incisions avoid rectal mucosa but can damage arteries.
4 After delivery, repair is carried out by a qualified midwife or obstetrician.

A: Accelerates difficult deliveries if there is maternal or fetal distress, ↓ pressure on the fetal head, ↓ incidence of damage to pelvic floor muscles and rectal mucosa/anal sphincter from a third degree tear. Episiotomy may be easier to repair than a ragged tear.

D: ↑ Incidence of haemorrhage, infection, perineal pain, dyspareunia, damage to Bartholin's gland (↓ vaginal lubrication and ↑ incidence of cyst) and damage to anal sphincter. Some women may see it as unnatural and prefer a natural tear.

C: Poor suturing can result in overtightening of the introitus resulting in pain and dyspareunia. This requires corrective surgery. Some evidence of more long-term complications (especially pain) with episiotomy than with laceration.

P: Excellent. Most heal very well. Those requiring corrective surgery at a later date usually have no further problems.

Evacuation of retained products of conception

D: Removal of any retained products of conception after delivery of the fetus (NB often normal with normal third stage), therapeutic abortion or miscarriage.

I: Incomplete placenta identified, inevitable miscarriage (if < 12 weeks), incomplete miscarriage, missed miscarriage (if < 12 weeks), incomplete therapeutic abortion, secondary post-partum haemorrhage.

M: **Prior to surgery:** Confirm presence of retained tissue with USS. NB Presence of a clot cannot be distinguished from a small piece of product of conception therefore the decision to evacuate primarily is a clinical one. If clinical evidence of sepsis, delay until parenteral antibiotics started. Provide broad-spectrum antibiotic cover (in all cases). Have cross-matched blood available.
Surgical Procedure: Anaesthetize and catheterize patient. Placed gloved hand into vagina and remove any clots, if bleeding starts again give Syntometrine IV. Dilate cervix slowly (if not already dilated), pass either index or middle finger through cervical canal into the uterus. Use free hand to press down on abdominal wall so that the whole uterine cavity can be examined and retained tissue loosened manually. Remove retained tissue using sponge forceps and suction evacuation. Experienced obstetrician required to carry out procedure if indication is secondary post-partum haemorrhage (high risk of perforation). Send any obtained tissues for histological examination.

A: Simple, quick procedure.
Prevents complications of retained products of conception.

D: Possibility of incomplete evacuation.
? Precludes possibility of spontaneous evacuation.

C: Uterine wall damage/perforation.
Haemorrhage.
Infection.
Dissemination of infection.
Asherman's syndrome (with sharp curettage).

P: Good.

External cephalic version

D: External manipulation of the fetus through the maternal abdomen in order to elicit a cephalic presentation.

I: Breech presentation, occasionally transverse.

M: Contraindicated with previous CS, myomectomy, placenta praevia, recent abruption, multiple pregnancy, pre-eclampsia. Prior to 32 weeks (primigravida) or 34 weeks (multigravida) either the fetus is likely to revert or the fetus may undergo spontaneous cephalic version.
Administer anti-D to Rhesus-negative patients. Carry out under tocolytic cover. Perform continuous fetal monitoring. Palpate to determine exact position. Knees bent position → ? facilitate relaxation of the abdominal muscles. Using manual pressure with both hands, disengage breech from pelvic brim. Then one hand used to push breech while other pushes head into direction which aids flexion. Steady pressure is used to convert fetus to cephalic presentation (→ an initially high presenting part).

A: ↓ Breech births.
↓ CS.

D: Little evidence to indicate whether CS or external cephalic version is best. Up to 50 % still require CS.
Not conclusively shown to improve fetal outcome.

C: Cord entanglement.
Retroplacental haemorrhage/placental abruption.
PROM.
Preterm labour.
Possible isoimmunization.
Scar dehiscence.

P: Roughly 50 % success rate.

IV infusion ritodrine 200 μg/min for 15 min
Scanning gel
rotate in direction — baby is facing
Check fetal HR every 2 min.
Give anti D 500 IU im

→ Leave breech rather than transverse if unsuccessful.

Fetal blood sampling in labour

D: Diagnostic test for fetal metabolic acidosis.

I: Suspected fetal distress, i.e. sustained tachycardia (HR > 160 bpm), variable decelerations (severe and prolonged dip), late decelerations, loss of variability.

M:
1. Mother placed in lithotomy position.
2. Amniotomy performed if needed.
3. Amnioscope (tubular speculum) inserted and fetal scalp sprayed with ethyl chloride to ↑ fetal blood flow.
4. Guarded blade is used to make small cut 2 mm deep.
5. Drop of blood is collected in a capillary tube (three separate samples preferable).
6. pH and base deficit is measured.
7. Further action depends on results of blood gas analysis. pH > 7.25 and base deficit < 6.0 mEq/L is normal and labour should be monitored as usual. pH 7.2–7.25 and base deficit 6.1–7.9 mEq/L indicates pre-asphyxia and if no other indications for delivery are present, e.g. fetal bradycardia, and delivery is imminent then labour should be allowed to continue under close supervision. If there is any deterioration then delivery should occur immediately. If not, repeat FBS after 30 min. pH < 7.2 and base deficit > 8.0 mEq/L indicates asphyxia and immediate delivery should occur by the most appropriate route.

A: May prevent unnecessary intervention as CTG is not always reliable. Only available test at present to confirm or exclude fetal hypoxia.

D: Small risk of scalp haemorrhage or infection. Discomfort to mother. Takes time. Contraindicated in HIV-positive, hepatitis B- or C-positive mothers, or if fetus suspected of having bleeding diathesis, e.g. thrombocytopaenia.

C: Rare. Include: **Fetal:** scalp haemorrhage, infection of wound. **Maternal:** Genital tract infection → puerperal pyrexia (see p. 77).

P: Fetal scalp pH correlates poorly with late Apgar scores. Outcome will depend on length of time fetus was deprived of oxygen.

Forceps delivery

D: Vaginal delivery assisted by the use of obstetric forceps.

I: Delayed progress of second stage labour (pelvic floor resistance, cephalo-pelvic disproportion, malpresentation (head), malpresentation, poor maternal effort, epidural).
Fetal distress/hypoxia.
Maternal distress, prevent extra maternal effort (underlying medical condition).
Preterm delivery (if very immature).
Breech presentation (aid delivery of head).

M: Check cervix fully dilated, membranes ruptured, head engaged, position known, bladder empty/catheterized.
Anaesthetize mother (pudendal/epidural/caudal), place in lithotomy position.
Select forceps type. *Long-shanked* (e.g. Neville–Barnes): if midcavity (head lies in pelvis at level of ischial spines). *Short-shanked* (e.g. Wrigley's): if low cavity (head below ischial spines) or outlet (head distends vaginal introitus). *Rotational* (e.g. Keilland's (very rarely used now due to risk of serious damage to mother or fetus. CS normally performed instead)): if midcavity with head not in direct occipitoanterior position.
  Insert left-hand blade along left side of vaginal wall supported by right cupped hand. Ensure correct position next to head and remove fingers. Repeat for right blade. Lock handles (should not be any resistance). Apply traction following pelvic curve.
? Episiotomy (if needed to prevent perineal tear).

A: Avoids CS.
Speeds up slow delivery.
Reduces maternal effort.

D: Skilled obstetrician required.
Severe lacerations if used incorrectly.
Failure to deliver possible.

C: **Maternal:** trauma (uterus, cervix, vagina, perineum), PPH, urinary retention, infection.
Fetal: bruising/cephalhaematoma, intracranial haemorrhage (incorrect application/excess traction), facial palsy (usually temporary), skull fracture.

P: Small risk of complications when procedure guidelines followed.

Hormone replacement therapy

- **D:** Oestrogen and progestogen (unopposed oestrogen →↑ risk endometrial carcinoma)—either cyclical (bleed regimens) or continuous combined (non-bleed regimens)/oestrogen only (previous hysterectomy), also tibolone (synthetic steroid with mild oestrogenic and progestogenic properties, non-bleed). Replacement usually used for 5–10 years.
- **I:** Menopausal women inconvenienced by vaginal atrophy/vasomotor symptoms, women with premature/iatrogenic menopause.
- **M:** Preparations: oral, transdermal patches/gel, subcutaneous implant.
- **A:** Symptomatic relief, prophylaxis against osteoporosis, cardiovascular disease, Alzheimer's.
- **D:** Withdrawal bleed/irregular bleed, premenstrual syndrome, weight gain, ↑ risk of breast cancer and thromboembolism.
- **C:** Recent history of oestrogen-dependant cancer, undiagnosed vaginal bleed, liver disease, venous thromboembolism.

Hysterectomy

D: Total hysterectomy is removal of the uterus and cervix. A subtotal hysterectomy is removal of the uterus but leaving the cervix. A radical hysterectomy with BSO and pelvic lympadenectomy is performed in cervical cancer. It includes removal of the uterus, fallopian tubes, ovaries, parametrium, upper third of the vagina and pelvic lymph nodes.

I: Fourth most common operative procedure in Western countries. Usually performed for menstrual disorders (fibroids, menorrhagia, PID, endometriosis, DUB), malignancy, dysmenorrhoea and prolapse.

M: May be performed abdominally (70 %) or vaginally (30 %). Laparoscopic hysterectomy is also used as an alternative to abdominal route.
Total abdominal hysterectomy (TAH): used in malignancy or if uterus is large and immobile (e.g. fibroids).
1 An incision is made through the abdomen, 2 cm above the pubic symphysis (just below the 'bikini line'), and the pelvic organs and vessels are exposed. Uterine and ovarian artery anastamoses are clamped, divided and tied. If BSO is being performed, the ovarian artery and vein is clamped, divided and tied instead. If fibroids are large or if malignancy is suspected a vertical incision is considered.
2 Uterine artery is clamped, divided and tied. Cardinal ligament is cut. Bladder is dissected off the cervix and vagina to prevent injury.
3 Cervicovaginal branches of the uterine artery are clamped, divided and tied. Uterosacral ligament is cut.
4 Uterus ± ovaries removed. Cervix may also be removed depending on reasons for hysterectomy.
Vaginal hysterectomy (VH): used mainly for prolapse or if uterus is relatively small and mobile. Similar method to that for TAH, but performed in reverse order, i.e. cervicovaginal branches divided first.
Laparoscopic hysterectomy (LH):
1 The uterine artery and veins are sealed off by diathermy, suture or staples under laparoscopic guidance.
2 The remainder of the procedure is then completed vaginally.
Radical hysterectomy: this is usually performed abdominally (Wertheim's hysterectomy) but occasionally is carried out vaginally (Schauta's hysterectomy).

A: Curative of gynaecological pathology (except malignant spread). Menstruation stops. LH enables removal of ovaries at same time (sometime difficult with VH), and ↓ scar tissue and recovery time. VH has lower morbidity than TAH. No risk of cervical cancer if cervix removed.

D: LH is a longer procedure so patient is under GA for longer time compared to VH and TAH. Patient is rendered infertile (if pre-menopausal).

C: **During procedure:** damage to ureters (↑ risk with LH), bladder or bowel, haemorrhage.
Acute complications: PE, infection (wound, chest, UTI), pelvic haematoma, urinary retention.
Long-term complications: menopausal symptoms if ovaries removed, psychosexual (may feel 'less' of a woman).

P: Depends on reason for procedure. Actual operation has 1 in 10 000 mortality rate.

Hysteroscopy

D: Visualization of the cervical canal and uterine cavity with a hysteroscope (fibreoptic telescope).

I: 1 Abnormal vaginal bleeding (including menorrhagia, irregular bleeding) in women >40 years or women <40 years who fail to respond to medical treatment.
2 Postmenopausal bleeding.
Also infertility problems; follow-up of uterine surgery; pelvic pain; foreign body removal; identification of endometrial polyps/carcinoma, uterine septa, fibroids.
Contraindicated in pregnancy, current pelvic infection, recent perforation.

M: **Preparation:** Carried out in outpatients or in theatre. Check for pregnancy in second half of cycle. ? Give mild analgesia. Patient placed in lithotomy position. Asepsis of vagina and cervix carried out. Local anaesthetic applied to cervix.
Procedure: Cervix dilated and hysteroscope placed in uterus. CO_2 or fluid is passed through and uterus distended. The uterine cavity is visualized and ? biopsies taken. Surgical procedures, e.g. fibroid removal, endometrial ablation and excision of septa, may be performed with prior cervical dilation via an operating hysteroscope (allows introduction of small surgical instruments/attachment of a camera to the instrument). ? Combined with laparoscopy for detection of uterine/tubal abnormalities/adhesions.

A: Non-surgical method of directly visualizing uterine cavity.
Avoids the need for preparation or anaesthesia.
Possibility of biopsy, and diagnosis.
Potential for surgical intervention—often with fast recovery.

D: ? Slight discomfort with introduction of scope and air/fluid.
? Slight discharge for a few weeks after the procedure.
As Complications.

C: Bleeding.
Infection.
Perforation.
Vasovagal shock.
Allergic reaction to the introduced solutions.
Air embolism.
Excessive leakage of introduced solution into peritoneal cavity/systemic circulation.
Spread of infection if present.
Danger to pregnancy if present.

P: Useful method of assessment and intervention. Complications rare.

Induction of labour

D: Artificial initiation of labour. 5–25% of labours are currently induced depending on centre.

I: **Maternal:** disease in danger of worsening with continued pregnancy, e.g. diabetes, cardiac disease, pre-eclampsia, poor obstetric history, fetal death, maternal request.
Fetal: post maturity (most common reason for induction in UK), IUGR, Rhesus sensitization (previous or current), fetal abnormality, APH, prolonged ROM (>24h).

M:
1. Assess cervical ripening using Bishops score which indicates probability of successful induction (see Table P.2). BS > 6 denotes favourable cervix and ↓ risk of complications/intervention.
2. If BS < 6 prime cervix with prostaglandins. Give 2 mg prostaglandin E2 pessary or gel into posterior fornix and reassess after 4 h.
3. If BS still < 6 repeat PGE$_2$ and reassess after 4 h. If < 6 repeat PGE$_2$ and reassess after 4 h. If no change consider CS.
4. If BS = 6 perform amniotomy. Observe for 1 h with continual CTG. If inefficient uterine contractions (< 3/10 min, duration < 45 s, mild pain, no cervical changes) give Syntocinon IV infusion and plot progress on partogram. If labour not progressing and delivery not imminent after 10 h following amniotomy, consider CS.

A: Minimizes complications that may be encountered with continued pregnancy. More 'natural' and less complications than with CS.

D: Contraindicated in acute fetal compromise, abnormal lie, placenta praevia, pelvic obstruction and > 1 previous CS. Has been reported to be more painful than spontaneous labour, so may require more analgesia. Less likely to be successful if < 34 weeks.

C: **Syntocinon:** uterine hyperstimulation → fetal distress, water intoxication (has ADH-like effect therefore must limit fluids), neonatal jaundice.
Amniotomy: intrauterine infection, cord prolapse.
Others: PPH (2 × greater risk), failure → CS.

P: Unsuccessful in 5% (1% if BS > 6 at first assessment).

Table P.2 Bishops score (BS) (maximum score = 10).

	Bishops score = 0	Bishops score = 1	Bishops score = 2
Dilation (cm)	0	1–2	>2
Length (cm)	>2	1–2	<1
Consistency	Firm	Medium	Soft
Position	Posterior	Central	Anterior
Station of head above iliac spines (cm)	3	2	1

Laparoscopy

D: Inspection of the pelvic organs with an endoscope.

I: **Diagnostic:** subfertility (inspect uterus, ovaries, tubes and tubal patency), chronic pelvic pain (unexplained), probable ectopic pregnancy, pelvic mass, endometriosis.
Therapeutic: endometriosis (cautery/laser ablation), adhesiolysis, ovarian cystectomy/cyst drainage, oophorectomy, sterilization (and reversal), upper vaginal hysterectomy, ventrosuspension.

M: Ensure patient has emptied bladder. Anaesthetize patient and place in Trendelenburg's position. Make small umbilical incision. Introduce a Veress needle and insufflate the abdominal cavity with 2–3 L of CO_2. Record intra-abdominal pressure, insert trocar then laparoscope. 1–2 additional instruments can be introduced through separate ports to facilitate surgery. Use abdominal pressure to expel CO_2 at end of procedure.

A: Allows investigation and treatment.
Better visualization of tissues.
↓ Tissue handling.
↓ Pain.
Faster postoperative recovery.
↓ Hospital inpatient stay (than laparotomy).

D: Invasive.
Requires GA.
Abdominal pain.
Visualization/treatment may be unsuccessful.

C: Complications of anaesthesia.
Damage to bowel, bladder, ureter or major blood vessels.
Haemorrhage.
Infection.
Surgical emphysema.
Incisional hernia.
Gas embolism.

P: Good, complications rare ($<5\%$), mortality very rare (<2 in 100 000).

Sterilization (female)

D: Surgical intervention intended to permanently prevent fertilization.

I: Desire for permanent contraception; situation where pregnancy would be undesirable or dangerous.

M: NB Preoperative counselling and explanation (both partners). Consider vasectomy as an alternative. Preoperative pregnancy testing. Advise continued use of contraception until operation and until next menstrual period following operation.
Tubal obstruction/ablation: generally carried out laparascopically by mini-laparotomy or at CS. Tubal occlusion using:
1 clips (Filshie/Hulka-Clemens);
2 occlusion rings (Fallope);
3 coagulation by diathermy.
Clips often preferred. Postpone operation for 6 weeks post pregnancy (↑ failure rate as difficult—large uterus, tubes high in abdomen—and tubes thicker).

A: Very reliable method of contraception, intended to be permanent.
↓ Incidence of unwanted pregnancy.
Immediately effective.
Low failure rate, <1%.

D: Possibility of regret.
Success rate of reversal variable (70% reported) but increased risk of tubal pregnancy (33%).
Failure (5 in 1000) sometimes not envisaged by patients.
May require laparotomy.
1% incidence chronic pain with diathermy sterilization.
Technically more difficult to perform than male sterilization.

C: Bruising, infection, pain.
Serious complications (mainly laparoscopy-related, e.g. bladder/bowel/vessel trauma) rare, ~1 in 200.
Risk bowel trauma/burns with diathermy sterilization.
Menstrual disorders reported ? cause.

P: Generally very effective. Clips easiest to reverse. ~1% seek reversal.

Therapeutic abortion

D: Termination of pregnancy by intervention.

I: May be performed in the UK under the conditions of the Abortion Act.
1 Continuing the pregnancy would involve a greater risk to the life of the pregnant woman than termination of the pregnancy.
2 Termination would prevent grave permanent injury to the physical or mental health of the pregnant woman.
3 The pregnancy has not exceeded 24 weeks and continuation would involve a greater risk to the pregnant woman's physical or mental health than termination.
4 The pregnancy has not exceeded 24 weeks and continuation would involve a greater risk to the health of any existing children than termination.
5 There is a substantial risk that if the child were born it would have a serious mental or physical handicap.

M: Counsel patient (options, procedures, advantages, disadvantages, support groups, ? partner support). Establish gestational length. *Bloods*: FBC, blood group, Rhesus status (if indicated).

Medical termination:
Mifepristone: (<6 weeks' gestation, also can be chosen between 7 and 9 weeks) Give mifepristone (antiprogesterone) 200–600 μg PO (as outpatient, stay on ward for 2 h in case vomits up), admit after 36–48 h and combine with prostaglandin:
Early: give prostaglandin vaginal pessary (Gemeprost 1 mg inserted into posterior fornix 3 h before surgery) *or* misoprostol 200–600 μg PO (can also be given as 800 μg PV). Confirm passage of conceptus.
Late: give prostaglandin as vaginal pessary (Gemeprost 1 mg inserted into posterior fornix every 3 h for a max. of 5 doses)/extra-amniotic infusion (through a balloon catheter passed through the cervix) or misoprostol PO (400 μg every 3 h up to 12 h), until fetus is delivered. Deliver placenta, check it is complete.
Keep on fluid diet (in case surgery required), fetus usually expelled in 4–6 h. 2 week follow-up.
NB Induction and vaginal delivery of fetus in late pregnancy (e.g. after injection of fetal heart to induce asystole).

Surgical termination:
Vacuum aspiration (early, <12 weeks gestation): give vaginal pessary prostaglandin. Anaesthetize patient. Dilate cervix (cervical dilator), introduce suction curette and aspirate uterine contents. Curette uterus to ensure it is empty (confirm with USS).
Piecemeal extraction (second trimester pregnancies): dilate cervix to 12–14 mm. Introduce crushing instruments to break up fetus before vacuum extraction.
EUA and ERPC (retained products of conception suspected): broad-spectrum antibiotic cover (doxycycline), anti-D (Rhesus-negative women).

A: ↓ Maternal mortality, short- and long-term maternal morbidity, morbidity of existent children.
Medical termination: avoids need for anaesthesia and surgery.
Surgical termination: quicker.

D: Possibility of procedure failure, psychological morbidity.
Medical termination: severe abdominal pain, longer period of blood loss.
Surgical termination: requires anaesthesia, invasive.

C: **Early:** haemorrhage, retained products of conception, infection, sepsis, uterine perforation, cervical laceration, isoimmunization.

Therapeutic abortion continued

Late: infertility, cervical incompetence, psychological morbidity.

P: Early (<12 weeks): <1 in 100 000 mortality, <1% complications.
Later (>12 weeks): 9–12 in 100 000 mortality, 3–5% complications.

Ultrasonography (in obstetrics and gynaecology)

D: Technique used to obtain images of internal anatomy, involving the transmission of pulsed ultrasound waves and the detection of reflected signals.

I: Gynaecology:
1 *Symptoms*: abnormal vaginal bleeding (IMB, PMB, menorrhagia), pelvic pain, pelvic mass, infertility.
2 *Suspected pathology*: uterus: fibroids, endometrial polyp, endometrial carcinoma; fallopian tubes: hydrosalpynx, pyosalpynx; ovary: PCOS, cyst, tumour, monitor ovulation.
3 *Therapeutic intervention*: ERPC, surgical TOP.

Obstetrics:
1 *Pregnancy confirmation*: from 6 weeks.
2 *Routine scans*: 11–14 weeks (gestational age, multiple gestation), 18–22 weeks (also ? abnormality, liquor volume, placenta position).
3 *Down's syndrome screening*: 10–12 weeks nuchal translucency.
4 *Clinical indication*. Early pregnancy: vaginal bleeding, abdominal pain; late pregnancy: vaginal bleeding, oligohydramnios, polyhydramnios, ? fetal movements. Suspected abnormality, early: ectopic pregnancy, trophoblastic disease, miscarriage/high risk of miscarriage; late: placenta praevia, malpresentation, IUGR—regular fetal monitoring, high risk of preterm labour.
5 *Guide invasive procedures*: diagnostic (amniocentesis, CVS, cordocentesis); therapeutic (fetal bladder shunt, chest drain).

M: Select scan type (abdominal/vaginal). Full bladder required for transabdominal scan. Cover transducer with film of gel and apply to abdomen/into vagina. Select image type static (1 μs pulse of ultrasound is directed through the body and the reflected echoes are detected in the following 1 ms)/'real time' (sequenced firing of transmitters and detection of echoes in rapid succession—20 × per s). Move transducer to obtain required image.
Gynaecology: inspect each pelvic organ. Note relevant measurements and pathological findings.
Obstetrics: check fetal growth, weight, anatomy, movement, position and presentation, placental location and morphology and amniotic fluid volume.

A: Relatively inexpensive, simple (used at bedside/as part of gynaecological examination), non-invasive, safe.
Transabdominal scan: not intrusive to patient.
Transvaginal scan: superior images, avoids need for full bladder.

D: Incorrect interpretation by operator possible. Poor image quality in obese patients.
Transabdominal scan: full bladder required.
Transvaginal scan: may be uncomfortable/intrusive to patient.

C: No known complications (evidence suggest it is safe for mother, fetus and operator).

P: n/a

Ventouse delivery

D: Instrumental delivery which involves an appropriate cup (silicone rubber, anterior metal or posterior metal) is attached to the fetal scalp by means of a vacuum suction. Traction is then applied by the obstetrician to facilitate delivery.

I: Prolonged second stage, fetal distress in second stage, maternal conditions requiring a short second stage.

M: Ensure full cervical dilation, fetal head engagement and good contractions.
1. The mother's perineum is infiltrated with 1% lignocaine (lidocaine).
2. An appropriate cup is inserted into the vagina sideways by pushing back against the perineum. The cup is placed on the vertex of the fetal scalp, being careful to exclude maternal vaginal wall and cervix.
3. A vacuum is created to a level of $0.8\,kg/cm^2$ and the connecting chain is pulled in synchrony with uterine contractions. The traction should be placed as vertical to the cup as possible in order to maintain suction. If the traction is too severe the vacuum is broken, thus avoiding excessive pull on the baby.
4. There should be significant descent of the fetus after three attempts which have been coordinated with uterine contractions. If there is no significant descent then alternative methods of delivery must be considered.

A: Mimics normal delivery and, unlike forceps, does not add to the width passing through the vagina so minimizes lacerations. Theoretically, can be used in skilled hands prior to full dilation, but has a high chance of being unsuccessful.

D: The ventouse can slip off. Delivery is longer with ventouse than forceps so is less useful in fetal distress. Baby has a very large caput and there is a high incidence of cephalohaematoma, resulting in an increased incidence of neonatal jaundice. Cup may cause lacerations to fetal scalp. The cosmetic damage to the infant's head can be distressing to the parents.

C: Contraindicated in face/breech presentation, <34 weeks' gestation, prolonged bleeding from fetal blood sampling site.

P: Failure rate (either CS or forceps required to deliver baby) is approx. 10–15% depending on indications, fetal head position, cup used and operator expertise.

APPENDICES

Antenatal care

PREPREGNANCY CARE
Advice: cessation of smoking, alcohol intake, rubella vaccination.
Folic acid supplementation 0.8 mg/day (↓ risk NTDs).
Ensure optimal management of pre-existing maternal disease (e.g. epilepsy, diabetes, etc.) and appropriate drug therapy.
Genetic counselling with family history of genetic disease.

ANTENATAL CARE
Types of care
Shared care: GP, community midwife and hospital consultant. Visits to the hospital for routine scans, booking and post-term visit or investigating problems. Care transferred to hospital for birth, back to GP and midwife post discharge.
Total consultant care: those with problems in previous pregnancies, those with pre-existing medical problems and at woman's request.
Midwifery care: midwife/team of midwives deliver baby in hospital/home. Responsible for antenatal and postnatal care.
Also: independent midwives/private consultant care.

Timing of visits
Differ depending on units, the following acts as a guide.
6–8 weeks: first GP visit—establish diagnosis. Advise about folic acid supplementation. Arrange booking visit.
8–12 weeks: hospital antenatal booking visit.
10–12 weeks: USS (dating scan and nuchal fold thickness for Down's syndrome).
16 weeks: biochemical screening.
18–20 weeks: scan for structural anomaly.
Routine appointments: every 4 weeks until 28 or 30 weeks → every 2 weeks until 36 weeks → weekly until full term.
34–40 week: scan in selected patients.
41 weeks: if prolonged pregnancy.

Antenatal booking visit
With both doctor and midwife.
History
Check medical history (diabetes, cardiac disease, epilepsy), surgical history (pelvic surgery), menstrual history (NB cycle length, recent OCP use to determine reliability of Naegele's rule), gynaecological history (PID, ectopic), obstetric history (previous operative delivery/difficult labour/labour complications, prematurity, pre-eclampsia, etc), social history, medication history, family history (genetic disease, twins), determine EDD—**Naegele's rule** (subtract 3 months from the first day of the last menstrual period and add 1 year and 7 days to that date).
Physical examination
General physical, baseline weight, BP. Examine respiratory and cardiovascular system. Examine abdomen for uterine size/fundal height, any abnormalities and auscultate for fetal heart sounds, If indicated, thorough examination of nervous and musculoskeletal systems.
Investigations
Routine tests: FBC (anaemia), blood group, Rhesus typing, anti-red cell antibodies (isoimmunization), rubella (? postnatal vaccination), hepatitis B (if positive → antenatal LFT, postnatal hepatology referral, vaccinate neonate), syphilis serology and MSU (? UTI).

Antenatal care continued

Certain groups: ? HIV, Hb electrophoresis (at-risk racial groups—sickle cell, thalassaemia), HVS (if high risk BV); hepatitis C (if blood transfusion before September 1991, history/partner history IV drug use), ? cervical smear if necessary.
Miscellaneous
Discuss with the woman the management of pregnancy, i.e. type of care, discuss antenatal classes and also discuss birth plan, noting any risk factors in labour.
Advise about diet (↑ protein, Ca, P, Fe; avoid liver—high vitamin A, unpasteurized foods—*Listeria*, raw eggs—*Salmonella*); social factors (alcohol, cigarettes, drugs, etc.); dental care.
Arrange dating scan.
? Fe supplementation (against anaemia) if inadequate/incomplete diet.

Dating scan
working environment → teratogenic?
+ flight attendant etc.
Dating via CRL measurement (up to 12 weeks' gestation and biparietal diameter thereafter, check for multiple pregnancy, viability, maternal reproductive pathology (e.g. fibroids/ovarian cysts if > 5 cm).

Subsequent antenatal appointments
Physical examination: BP; ? weight—probably only useful at first visit and in late pregnancy; abdominal palpation—fundal height, auscultate FHR, after 36 weeks assess engagement of head; check for swelling, especially fingers/face (pre-eclampsia).
Investigations: MSU (? protein/glucose); 30 and 36 weeks check FBC (anaemia).
Advice: breast care, ? fetal movement counting from 32 weeks if monitoring required.
41 weeks: assess as for routine appointments; also fetal assessment with USS/CTG; consider induction.
NB Anti-D administration for Rhesus-negative women at 28–34 weeks (see p. 78).

Testing in later gestation
Serum markers (NTDs, trisomy 21): maternal choice, e.g. triple/double marker test (∼16 weeks) produces numerical risk for Down's, > 1 in 300 → high risk (↓ AFP, ↓ unconjugated oestriol, ↑ hCG in association with ↑ age → increased risk).
Anomaly scan (structural abnormalities, infection and aneuploidy markers): examine skull, face, chest and diaphragm, spinal column, stomach, liver, liquor volume, placenta, cerebral ventricles, cerebellum, cisterna magna, eyes, heart, limbs, urinary system, cord insertion, fetal behaviour, serial for fetal growth.
Prenatal diagnosis: if appropriate.
Timing of prenatal diagnosis:
CVS 10+ weeks
Amniocentesis 15+ weeks
Cordocentesis 20+ weeks

Antenatal care continued

Antenatal classes
Last trimester
Discuss changes in late pregnancy, labour (e.g. procedure, analgesia), exercises during pregnancy, posture, feeding, etc.

Contraception

$$\text{Pearl index (PI)} = \frac{\text{number of pregnancies}}{\text{number of couples having intercourse}} \times 100 \text{ women/year}$$

NATURAL METHODS
Mechanism (M):
1 *Rhythm*: avoids fertile period by observing body temperature (? 0.2 °C preovulation, ? 0.5 °C in luteal phase), cervical secretions (ferning and spinnbarkeit (elastic strings) indicate fertile period) and length of cycle.
2 *Withdrawal*: removal of penis before ejaculation.
3 *Lactation*.
4 *Persona*: special kit available from chemists which measures daily concentration of hormones in woman's urine to determine when fertile period is.
Efficacy (E): poor.
Advantages (A): no barrier method/hormones, cheap, acceptable.
Disadvantages (D): least reliable method, only effective if used correctly therefore requires commitment, no sexually transmitted disease protection, withdrawal interrupts intercourse.

BARRIER METHODS
Male (condom)
M Rubber sheath fits over erect penis.
E PI = 3.5.
A Non-hormonal, STI protection, cheap (obtained free from family planning clinics).
D Inconvenient, unreliable if used incorrectly, need to withdraw as soon as ejaculated.

Female (condoms, diaphragm and cap)
M Diaphragm and cap (cap smaller than diaphragm) fit over cervix and left in for 8 h after intercourse (used with spermicide). Female condom is a larger version of the male condom inserted into the vagina with two rings which aid positioning.
E PI = 20.
A Non-hormonal, limited sexually transmitted disease protection, cheap.
D Interrupts intercourse, ↑ cystitis, annual fitting check with cap/diaphragm (less effective if change > 3.5 kg in weight, childbirth, abortion).

COMBINED ORAL CONTRACEPTIVE PILL
M Suppresses ovulation by ↓ GnRH (oestrogen ↓ FSH, progesterone inhibits LH surge), makes endometrium inhospitable, thickens cervical mucus. Monophasic pills (e.g. Loestrin, Microgynon) give continuous oestrogen and progesterone for 21 days followed by 7-day break, biphasic pills (e.g. BiNovum) give continuous oestrogen and low-dose progesterone for 7 days, then higher dose for 14 days followed by 7-day break while triphasic pills (e.g. Tri-Minulet) provide three different doses of oestrogen and progesterone over 21 days, e.g. Tri-Minulet provides 30 μg of oestrogen and 50 μg of progesterone for the first 6 days, followed by 40 μg oestrogen and 70 μg progesterone for the next 5 days and finally 30 μg oestrogen and 100 μg of progesterone for the last 10 days. This helps to prevent breakthrough bleeding. During the 7-day break a withdrawal bleed occurs (not a period). Placebo tablets may be taken to help compliance.
E PI = < 0.2.

Contraception continued

A Highly effective, ↓ menstrual problems (triphasic may give better cycle control), benign breast disease, ovarian cysts, fibroids, PID, endometrial and ovarian cancer.
D Side-effects: *Circulation*: DVT, PE, MI, CVA, arterial thrombosis (? risk with third-generation progesterone containing pills, e.g. Marvelon compared to second-generation progesterone pills: 3 in 10 000 as opposed to 2 in 10 000). *Malignancy*: ? ↑ breast and cervical cancer. *Liver*: adenoma, hepatocellular carcinoma, cholestatic jaundice. *Other*: fluid retention, ↑ weight (introduction of new pill, Yasmin, has been shown to avoid this and may even promote slight weight loss), impaired glucose tolerance, breakthrough bleeding, worsening of migraine.
Contraindicated: *Absolute*: history of DVT, CVA, IHD, TIA, cholestatic jaundice on COC pill/pregnancy, severe focal migraine with aura, presence of oestrogen-dependent tumour, blood clotting defects, history of thrombophilia, pregnancy, smokers >35 years, active/chronic liver disease, gallstones, hypertension, hyperlipidaemia. *Relative*: smokers, obesity, diabetes, renal disease, >40 years, sickle cell disease, postnatal.
Advice: educate on symptoms to look out for. First pill taken on first day of period, or second day after miscarriage or TOP. ↓ Absorption with diarrhoea and vomiting, and certain antibiotics (e.g. tetracycline) → use alternative method for 1 week. Drug interactions (e.g. ↑ dose required if on anticonvulsants). Missed pill: if <12 h—take as soon as possible; if >12 h take as soon as possible and use alternative methods of contraception for 1 week; if <7 days until end of packet, continue with next packet without 7-day break. Regular check ups required (BP, glycosuria and excessive weight gain). NB It is safe to take up to four packets continuously.

PROGESTERONE ONLY PILL
M Thickens cervical mucus, endometrium inhospitable, ↓ tubal motility, inhibits ovulation in ≤50%. Taken continuously (each pill must be taken at same time each day ±2 h).
E PI = 1.0.
A No oestrogen-dependent risks, can be taken when lactating as does not affect milk production, ↓ progesterone dose than COC pill.
D Irregular bleeding, ↑ weight, headaches, depression, ↑ ectopic pregnancy if conceived while taking pill, ↑ functional cysts, must be taken at same time each day (new POP currently in trials has a 12-h window).
Advice: if >2 h late taking pill, use alternative method for 14 days.

INJECTION
M Progesterone IM injection every 3 months (Depo-Provera).
E PI = <1.0.
A Easy to comply with, ? menstrual problems.
D Progesterone side-effects (have to wait 3 months before side-effects wear off).

COIL (IUCD/IUS (MIRENA))
M *IUCD*: usually contains copper (e.g. Multiload, Nova-T). Prevents implantation. Copper also spermicidal and bactericidal. *IUS*: Mirena is most common form of coil currently inserted in UK. Produces local slow release of progesterone (levonorgestrel). Coil inserted at end of period, 6 weeks postnatally or following TOP.
E *IUCD*: PI = 2.0. *IUS*: PI = <0.1.

Contraception continued

A 'Fit and forget', safe, can be used as emergency contraception if put in within 5 days of intercourse. *Mirena* ↓ menstrual loss (50 % amenorrhoea).
D *On insertion*: cervical shock (↑ vagal tone), perforation (1 in 500), expulsion (usually within first month). *IUCD*: menorrhagia, ↑ PID, ↑ ectopic if conception occurs while IUCD in place. *IUS*: slightly bigger than copper devices, therefore may be more difficult to insert especially in nulliparous women, ↑ ectopic.
Advice: on insertion screen for existing STIs and give antibiotic cover for 7 days. Advise to check for string after each period. Change after 5 years.

EMERGENCY CONTRACEPTION
Morning after pill: 75 μg levonorgestrel or 100 μg ethinylestradiol + 250 μg levonorgestrel taken within 72 h of intercourse and repeated 12 h later.
IUCD: See coil.

RECENT/FUTURE ADVANCEMENTS
Vaginal ring: ring placed in vagina, providing local release of hormones, which is removed after 3 weeks, when withdrawal bleed will occur and replaced after 7 days.
Hormone patches: sticky patches containing hormones are used for 3 weeks and then removed for withdrawal bleed.
Implanon: subdermal rod containing etonogestrel is inserted into lower surface of upper arm. Effective for 3 years.
New pill advancements: *Yasmin*: contains drospirenone (new type of progestogen that has mild diuretic activity). Advantages include reduced incidence of hypertension, weight gain, mood swings and fluid retention. Disadvantages include cost and raised potassium levels in those with renal, hepatic or adrenal impairment. *Seasonale*: combined pill taken continuously for 84 days, resulting in only 4 withdrawal bleeds per year. *Cerazette*: POP which reliably stops ovulation, has a regulating effect on menstruation and has a 12-h window period in which it can be taken, unlike the 2-h period of traditional POP.

Drugs in pregnancy

Only prescribe drugs during pregnancy if the benefits to the mother are greater than any expected risks to the fetus. Drugs may potentially affect the fetus at any stage of pregnancy. The following can be affected (Table A.1):
1 *organogenesis* (first trimester): to produce congenital malformations (teratogenesis);
2 *growth and development* (> day 56);
3 *neonate*: if given at the end of pregnancy.

Drug class	Drug	Risk to organogenesis (O), growth + development (GD) or neonate (N) / Advise
Antiarrhythmics	Amiodarone	GD/N: neonatal goitre, hypothyroidism. **CI** (use only if no alternative)
Antibiotics	Aminoglycosides	GD: auditory/vesticular nerve damage. **Avoid**
	Chloramphenicol	N: neonatal 'grey syndrome'. **CI**
	Metronidazole	O: **Avoid** GD/N: **Avoid** high dose regimens/ prolonged use
	Sulphonamides	N: Neonatal haemolysis, methaemoglobinaemia. **Caution**
	Tetracyclines	GD/N: dental discoloration
	Trimethoprim	O: limb reduction, cleft palate. **Caution**
Anticoagulants	Warfarin	O: congenital malformations GD/N: fetal and neonatal haemorrhage. **CI**
Antidepressants		Only use if potential benefits outweigh risks
	Tricyclic antidepressants	N: low risks of tachycardia, irritability, muscle spasms. Less information available on other groups. **Caution**
Antiepileptics	Carbamazepine, phenobarbital, phenytoin, sodium valproate, vigabatrin	Benefit of treatment outweighs risks. O: teratogenicity including NTDs (folate deficiency) GD/N: bleeding (vitamin K deficiency)
Antifungals	Fluconazole	O: multiple congenital abnormalities. **Caution**
Antihypertensives/ cardiac drugs	ACE inhibitors	O: skull defects GD/N: may adversely affect fetal and neonatal BP and renal function. **Avoid**

Drugs in pregnancy continued

Table A.1 continued

Drug class	Drug	Risk to organogenesis (O), growth + development (GD) or neonate (N) / Advise
	β-blockers	GD/N: may cause IUGR, neonatal hypoglycaemia, bradycardia. Maternal hypertension is a greater risk
Antimalarials		Benefit of prophylaxis and treatment of malaria outweighs risk. Chloroquine preferred for prophylaxis and treatment
	Primaquine	GD/N: neonatal haemolysis, methaemoglobinaemia, Postpone treatment until after pregnancy, use chloroquine in interim. **Caution**
	Proguanil	O: teratogen unless folate supplements provided. **Caution**
Antimanics	Lithium	O: teratogenecity, cardiac anomalies N: toxicity. **Caution**
Antimitotics	Podophyllum resin	O: teratogenesis N: neonatal death. **CI**
	Podophyllotoxin	CI
Antipsychotics		N: extrapyramidal effects.
	Carbamazepine, phenobarbital	O: teratogenicity—give folate supplements with Carbamazepine N: bleeding. **Caution**
Antithyroids	Carbimazole, iodide, iodine	N: goitre and hypothyroidism. **Caution**
	Radioactive iodide	Permanent hypothyroidism. **CI**
Antivirals	Ganciclovir	O: teratogenesis. **CI**
Biguanides	Metformin	Can provoke maternal lactic acidosis. **Avoid.** Substitute insulin.
Bronchodilators	Theophylline	N: irritability, apnoea. **Caution**
Diuretics	Thiazides	N: Thrombocytopenia. **Caution**
Fibrinolytics	Streptokinase	GD: premature placental separation, theoretical risk of haemorrhage
General anaesthetics		O: teratogenic risk from hypoxia N: respiratory depression

Drugs in pregnancy continued

Gonadotrophin inhibitors	Danazol	GD/N: weak androgenic effects and virilization of the female fetus. **CI**
Local anaesthetics		N: respiratory depression, bradycardia, hypotonia, with large doses after epidural or paracervical block
Lipid lowering	Statins	O: congenital anomalies. **CI**
NSAIDs		GD/N: premature closure of the ductus arteriosus, persistent pulmonary hypertension, delayed and prolonged labour. **Avoid**
	Aspirin	GD/N: impaired platelet function, haemorrhage. **CI**
Opioids		N: respiratory depression, dependency and irritability, (NB If mother dependent withdraw slowly). **Caution**
Retinoids	Isotretinoin, tretinoin	O: teratogenic (use effective contraception). **CI**
Sex hormones: Anabolic steroids, androgens		O/GD/N: masculinization of female fetus. **CI**
Oestrogens	Diethylstilbestrol	Increased risk of vaginal carcinoma, urogenital abnormalities and reduced fertility in female offspring if high doses used. **Avoid**
Progestogens	Hydroxy-progesterone, medroxyprog-esterone acetate	O: genital malformations. **Caution** O: genital malformations. **CI**
Sulphonylureas		N: neonatal hypoglycaemia. Substitute insulin/stop 2 days before delivery
Tranquilizers	Barbiturates	N: withdrawal effects. **CI**
	Benzodiazepines	N: withdrawal effects, neonatal hypothermia, hypotonia, respiratory depression. Avoid regular use. **Caution**

Infections in pregnancy

A baby's immune system is not fully developed until well after birth. The fetus produces no IgM until >20 weeks' gestation, while maternal IgG may persist in the infant's blood for many months following birth. Any maternal infection during pregnancy can have implications for the fetus, especially if the mother suffers with a high fever, but there are certain infections that carry specific risk especially if they are able to cross the placenta.

These are:
Rubella
CMV
Varicella zoster
HIV
Hepatitis B
Toxoplasma
Listeria
Chlamydia
Parvo virus B19
Syphilis

RUBELLA

Epidemiology (E): Rare, as 97% of women in UK are immune as a result of rubella immunization at 11–13 years.

Route of transmission (Ro): Person–person spread. Incubation period is 14–21 days, patient is infectious from 7 days before onset of rash to 4 days after rash has appeared.

Risk of transmission to fetus (R): Primary maternal infection during first 12 weeks' gestation results in fetal transmission in ≤95% of cases. Incidence of severe damage depends on gestational age at time of infection and may be as high as 90% if <8 weeks. Risk of severe complications ↓ with advancing gestational age.

Maternal effects (M): Mild fever and maculopapular rash but may be asymptomatic. Risk of damage to fetus is unrelated to severity of maternal infection therefore diagnosis is often missed.

Fetal effects (F): Classical triad of damage is blindness, deafness and cardiac malformation (VSD, PDA). Other complications include hepatosplenomegaly, jaundice and microcephaly, cerebral palsy and thrombocytopaenia.

Investigations (I): Suspect rubella infection in any small for dates baby with congenital abnormality including microcephaly and hepatosplenomegaly. Blood test based on detection of 4 × ↑ in IgG antibodies in serum of mother or child 28 days post exposure. IgM in fetal blood (from fetal blood sample) >22 weeks indicates fetal transmission.

Treatment (T): Counselling regarding TOP if infection <12 weeks' gestation.

Prevention (P): Non-pregnant women who are not immune to rubella may be offered vaccine (avoid in pregnancy). Since 1988, MMR is offered to all children from 15 to 18 months and a follow-up booster is given at school entry. Recent concerns about use of MMR in children have led to ↓ uptake and therefore ↑ risk of susceptible women in the future.

Infections in pregnancy continued

CYTOMEGALOVIRUS (MEMBER OF HERPES FAMILY)
E 1200 babies born per annum in the UK with congenital CMV. 50–70 % of pregnant women are at risk. The higher the socioeconomic class the more at risk as women in this group are less likely to have acquired the virus as a child.
Ro Person–person spread.
R 1 % of women become infected during pregnancy. Primary maternal infection in pregnancy results in 40 % fetal transmission. 90 % of these are normal at birth, and of these 20 % will experience long-term problems. Reactivation of CMV has < 1 % transmission rate to fetus.
M Usually asymptomatic.
F Microcephaly, blindness, deafness, liver dysfunction, pneumonitis, chorioretinitis and mental retardation. Infection is more serious if acquired later in pregnancy.
I Maternal IgM and IgG elevation. PCR on amniotic fluid can be performed but not accurate (45 % false-positives)
T Difficult to treat before birth as no accurate test to prove infection. TOP not recommended.
P No vaccine available.

VARICELLA ZOSTER (MEMBER OF HERPES FAMILY)   (Ig M in mat serum indicates 1° varicella)
E 85 % of women are immune, and although primary infection is not uncommon, it is not usually a problem.
Ro Spread via respiratory route. Very infectious. Incubation period is 10–20 days.
R Infection in late pregnancy, i.e. < 7 days before delivery is more of a problem as the baby may be born infected before the mother has had time to produce the antibodies which could be passed to the fetus as passive immunity. Infection in first trimester causes congenital abnormalities (risk < 2 %).
M Intensely itchy papules and pustules on the skin. Malaise. ? Risk (10 %) of varicella pneumonia in pregnancy (cause of maternal mortality prior to availability of aciclovir).
F Can lead to congenital varicella syndrome if infection occurs in first trimester; dermal and skeletal scarring, hypoplasia of the limb bones, muscular atrophy, chorioretinitis, cataracts and cerebral atrophy. *Neonate*: at risk of neonatal varicella which has a 30 % mortality if untreated.
T If mother unwell with infection admit to hospital and give aciclovir. Varicella zoster immunoglobulin given in following circumstances:
1 to mother if < 10 days from contact;
2 to neonate if mother develops infection 7 days before to 28 days after delivery, if in contact with chickenpox and mother has no previous history of infection *or* if baby < 30 weeks and in contact with infection, regardless of mother's history.
This reduces the mortality rate to almost zero.

HIV
E 0.6 % of women in inner cities in the UK. ↑ Prevalence in sub-Saharan Africa and South and South East Asia.
Ro Transmitted by blood or body fluid of infected person.

Infections in pregnancy continued

R Vertical transmission is 15%. ↑ Risk with ↓ CD4 count ↑ viral load, breastfeeding (especially when seroconverting) and prolonged ROM (>4h).
M Usually asymptomatic in latent phase (8–10 years). May have initial febrile seroconversion illness. In later stages may get opportunistic infections, e.g. recurrent *Candida*, genital herpes. No evidence that pregnancy ↑ progression to AIDS.
F Stillbirth and IUGR. Almost half of infected neonates will have AIDS by 5 years.
I Screening available on request. Routinely offered in some parts of UK, e.g. London. For HIV-positive, monitor CD4 count and viral load.
T/P In UK: Zidovudine 100 mg PO 5 × per day started between 14 and 34 weeks and is continued throughout labour as continuous infusion. Given to neonate for 6 weeks post delivery. Minimize risk of contact of fetus with maternal bodily fluids, i.e. offer CS. If vaginal delivery, avoid prolonged ROM, instrumental delivery, fetal blood sampling etc. Avoid breastfeeding.

HEPATITIS B
E Prevalence varies according to population, common in parts of Africa, East and South East Asia and Mediterranean countries.
Ro Transmitted by blood or body fluid contact of infected person.
R ↑ Risk of transmission with HBcAG and HBsAG present in blood (up to 90% transmission rate) or if HBeAG-positive and HBeAB-negative. Presence of HBeAG indicates high infectivity. ↓ Transmission with presence of HBeAB (10%).
M Acute infection causes acute hepatitis, and in severe cases fulminating hepatic failure (1% of infected patients). Some patients may develop chronic disease (chronic active hepatitis, cirrhosis and ↑ risk of hepatocellular carcinoma).
F Neonatal hepatitis (significant mortality).
I Most units now screen all women. High-risk women include immigrants (especially from parts of Africa, East and South East Asia, Mediterranean countries), those born or childhood outside the UK, IV drug users and people with a high number of sexual partners. Tests for infection include HBsAg, HBeAg and anti-HBcAgIgM.
T/P All babies whose mothers are carriers should be treated to prevent vertical transmission. If the mother only carries antibodies, the baby should be vaccinated at birth, 1 month and 6 months. If the mother has antigen in her blood, the baby must be given hepatitis B immunglobulin in addition to the vaccine within 12 h of birth.

TOXOPLASMOSIS (*TOXOPLASMA GONDII*)
E 1 in 500 women acquire toxoplasmosis during pregnancy but fetal infection rate is far less. 1 in 60 000 babies born with signs of toxoplasma infection. In the UK, 15% of women are immune because of prior infection before becoming pregnant, whereas in France 90% of women are immune. Despite low immunity the chances of acquiring the infection during pregnancy are low (0.2%).
Ro Contact with cat faeces and eating infected meat.
R Transmission rate is 20% in the first trimester, 80% in third. Risk of fetal damage from infection ? from 60% in the first trimester to almost 0% at term.
M Incubation period 2 days. Majority asymptomatic. Occasionally mild rash or lymphadenopathy.

Infections in pregnancy continued

F Eyes and central nervous system most often affected. Triad of fetal damage is hydrocephaly, retinochoroiditis and intracranial calcification. Other features include miscarriage, IUGR, convulsions, thrombocytopaenia, hepatosplenomegaly.
I Recent infection in women in early pregnancy can be detected using specific IgM tests, although these are not 100 % reliable.
T Counsel about TOP only if infected < 20 weeks. If infection proven give spiramycin.
P Avoid handling cat faeces and touching eyes/mouth after handling raw meat. Avoid eating raw meat and unwashed fruit and vegetables.

LISTERIOSIS (*LISTERIA MONOCYTOGENES*)
E Incidence 1 in 20 000 pregnancies in the UK.
Ro This Gram-positive coccobacillus can live non-pathologically in the bowel of 10 % of the normal population. It is caught from refrigerated faecally contaminated foods, e.g. unpasteurized coleslaw, paté and soft cheese.
R Transmission to fetus results from bacteraemia in pregnancy (0.01 % of women).
M Gastroenteritis, non-specific, 'flu-like illness possibly with backache and fever. It can give rise to systemic infection which, if it coincides with early pregnancy, can cause miscarriage or, if acquired later, premature labour.
F Infection with *Listeria* should be thought of if meconium is passed by the premature baby. May result in respiratory distress and a petechial rash. Perinatal infection can cause pneumonia, meningitis and septicaemia and may occur 2–5 weeks after delivery. Mortality from established infection is high.
I Swab from throat/genital tract of mother, blood culture or culture of liquor or placenta.
T Amoxicillin and gentamicin.
P Avoid high-risk food.

CHLAMYDIA
E Infection in pregnancy occurs in ∼ 5 % of women.
Ro STI. Transmitted to fetus via ascending infection and during delivery.
M See p. 25
F Prematurity, neonatal conjunctivitis, pneumonitis.
I Investigations of suspected ocular infection in the neonate should be swabs from the eye, nasopharynx and throat. Endocervical swabs from mother.
T Chlortetracycline eye drops. Tetracycline should not be given to either pregnant women or neonates because of discoloration of teeth. If systemic treatment required give oral erythromycin. If *Chlamydia* is detected in the mother in pregnancy, treatment is 500 mg erythromycin 4 × per day for 7 days.

PARVO VIRUS B19 (ERYTHEMA INFECTIOSUM OR FIFTH DISEASE)
E 50 % of women immune. Affects 0.25 % of pregnant women.
Ro Respiratory route (usually from children). Incubation period of 4–20 days.
R 30 % transmission rate if < 20 weeks.
M May be asymptomatic, or 'slapped cheek' appearance.

Infections in pregnancy continued

F Usually before 20 weeks: aplastic anaemia, hydrops fetalis, myocarditis, fetal death (10 % infected fetuses).
I ↑ Maternal IgM with symptoms, followed by ↑ IgG after 1 week. Fetal diagnosis made by PCR of fetal blood sample.
T *In utero* blood transfusion if evidence of cardiac failure.

SYPHILIS
E Rare, <0.1 %
Ro STI. *Treponema pallidum* are able to pass across the placenta after 15 weeks.
F Fetal death, congenital syphilis.
I Every pregnant woman screened at booking with either an ELISA, VDRL or rapid plasma reagin test. If positive, clarify (as false-positives occur) with antitreponemal antibody test, e.g. TPHA.
T Penicillin.

β haemolytic streptococci - group B.
- 5-20% woman carry in vagina
- 1% develop infection @ birth
- 80% mortality
- 50% of these survive meningitis
- give amoxicillin intrapartum

Intrapartum care

Aim: to deliver healthy baby to healthy mother by ensuring maternal and fetal well-being and progress during labour.

ON ADMISSION
Admit when contractions are every 10 min and/or membranes ruptured.
1 Short history of pregnancy.
2 Determine labour has started: (i) regular, painful contractions; (ii) cervical dilation and effacement ± 'show'.
3 Begin partogram (monitors strength, duration and frequency of contraction, cervical effacement and dilation, station (descent of fetal head), FHR, maternal well-being (BP, HR, temperature) and liquor (blood-/meconium-stained).
4 Offer shower and encourage to empty bowel.

FIRST STAGE
First stage is from onset of labour to full cervical dilation. Onset of labour is difficult to determine by contractions alone (Braxton–Hicks contractions are normal after 30th week = tight, palpable, painless contractions)—usually defined as cervical dilatation >2 cm in presence of painful contractions occurring >10 mins.

Divided into *latent phase* (during effacement, dilation <3 cm) and *active phase* (dilation ≥3 cm). Takes an average of 8 h in primigravida and 5.5 h in multigravida.
1 *Monitor labour progression*: by plotting changes on partogram every 2 h. Abnormal progress if dilating <1 cm/h in active phase, or if first stage >12 h.
2 *Ensure maternal well-being*: partner support, light snacks and fluids, encourage frequent passing of urine.
3 *Offer analgesia.* (i) *Non-pharmacological*: TENS machine, warm bath, back massage, relaxation techniques. (ii) *Entonox*: 50:50 mixture of nitrous oxide and oxygen. Given via mouthpiece or mask with contractions in first stage and during second stage. Mild analgesic with rapid onset, but fails to provide adequate pain relief in ≥50% of women. Side-effects include nausea, vomiting, dizziness, hyperventilation, light headedness. (iii) *Opiates*: pethidine or diamorphine depending on centre. Given IM during labour when patient requests, but preferably >2 h before delivery because of risk of respiratory distress in newborn. Onset within 25 min, effects last ≤4 h. ↓ Awareness of pain, so patient less concerned. Side-effects: nausea, vomiting, ? gastric emptying, drowsiness, confusion, feels out of control, respiratory distress in newborn. (iv) *Epidural* (see p. 105)
4 *Ensure fetal well-being*: FH every 15 min with hand-held Doppler or fetal stethoscope and 20-min CTG every 2 h in low risk, continual CTG in high risk, monitor liquor.

SECOND STAGE
Second stage is from full cervical dilation to delivery of fetus.

Divided into *passive stage* which lasts for 1 h (increased to 2 h if epidural used) during which no active encouragement to push, and *active stage* when the mother is encouraged to push. Lasts for 1 h. If >1 h, intervention is usually needed (ventouse/forceps) as a result of maternal exhaustion.

Intrapartum care continued

1 Ensure attendant constantly present when fully dilated.
2 During active stage encourage pushing with each contraction (deep breath, chin on chest and bear down). Aim for three pushes per contraction.
3 When ~5 cm of fetal head is visible between labia, attendant scrubs and gowns.
4 During each contraction the fetal head is flexed by index finger of left hand, while protecting the perineum with a pad. When the head crowns (i.e. widest part—biparietal diameter—has passed through the introitus, no retraction of head between contractions) mother stops pushing and pants to allow controlled delivery of the head to minimize trauma. Episiotomy performed prior to crowning if indicated (see p. 106).
5 Attendant's left hand then flexes head, while right hand pushes chin up to encourage extension as head passes through perineum.
6 When head is born, allow a few seconds for restitution to occur (rotates 90°) and check neck to ensure cord is not wrapped around it.
7 With next contraction, head is held with both hands and pulled gently posteriorly to deliver anterior shoulder. Syntometrine/Syntocinon is given if indicated (see below). Head is then pulled anteriorly to deliver posterior shoulder.
8 Body and legs are delivered, baby suctioned and given to mother. Cord clamped and cut after 2–3 min.

THIRD STAGE
Third stage is from delivery of fetus to delivery of placenta.

Traditional management
1 Await signs of placental separation (lengthening of cord, rising and narrowing of uterine fundus, gush of blood). Average time is 10–20 min.
2 Rub up uterine contraction.
3 Contracted uterus pushed down towards pelvis to aid expulsion of placenta.

Active management
1 Syntometrine or Syntocinon (if ↑ BP) given IM following delivery of anterior shoulder to produce a uterine contraction.
2 When uterine contraction felt after delivery, *Brandt–Andrews* method is used to deliver placenta (left hand placed suprapubically and pushes uterus 'upwards' while right hand grasps cord and gently pulls placenta out of vagina).
  Placenta, cord and membranes are examined to check for completeness and any abnormalities. Advantages of active management are ↓ average length of third stage and ↓ incidence of PPH (from 4 % with traditional management to 1 % with active management). Disadvantage is ↑ incidence of uterine inversion if managed incorrectly.

Postnatal care

EXAMINATION OF THE NEWBORN POST DELIVERY
Assess Apgar score at 1 and 5 min (see Table A.2).
Record: weight, temperature, sex, passage of urine/meconium, cord blood pH/base excess.
Inspect: general appearance (? structural abnormality, appearance of syndrome); also for moulding, marks from instrumental delivery, skin (intact, birthmarks, etc.), presence of eyes, cleft palate, digits, spine (? straight, ? sacral dimples), testicular descent, hips (developmental dysplastic hip).

HOSPITAL CARE POST DELIVERY
Neonate
Blood type from cord blood. NB administer anti-D if neonate Rh-positive and mother Rh-negative (? Kleihauer test necessary).
Paediatric examination within 24 h.
Ensure identification bands are applied.

Mother
Examination: ? signs of anaemia, temperature (puerperal sepsis. NB often raised temporarily for 24 h with epidural); BP (? pre-eclampsia, hypotension); abdomen (bladder emptying, uterine fundus for involution); episiotomy wound; surgical scars; legs (DVT); ? breast exam.
Assess maternal mood; ensure passage of urine; enquire about lochia.
Advice: contraception (no COC if lactating), breastfeeding (positioning, timing. NB should occur within 1 h post delivery), breast care, vulval hygiene (cover with sterile pad, change regularly), caution against bladder overdistention ($\downarrow$ sensation, emptying and antidiuretic oxytocin). NB pain relief. Discharge after at least 6 h post hospital delivery.

WARD CARE POST CAESAREAN SECTION
Regular (1/2 hourly) observations + assess lochial loss and wound.
Watch bladder emptying, avoid overdistension, catheter for first 24 h.
Monitor: pain control, fluid balance.
Encourage mobilization within 24 h.
Admit for average 6 days, review day 1, full postnatal check day 2, days 3–5 assess bowel movement and lochia, suture removal days 5–6.
Check FBC.

Table A.2 Apgar scoring system.

	0	1	2
Skin colour	Pale/blue	Pink body, pale limbs	Pink
Heart rate	Absent	<100 bpm	>100 bpm
Response	Absent	Facial grimace	Crying
Muscle tone	Limp	Some flexion	Active movement
Respiratory effort	Absent	Slow to cry	Strong cry

Postnatal care continued

COMMUNITY CARE POST DISCHARGE

Legal requirement for daily midwife contact/consultation for at least 10 days post delivery.

6-week postnatal health check undertaken by GP.

1 Debriefing of pregnancy/labour (? complicated/unexpected outcome) and ? plans for future pregnancies.

2 Assess: general health; whether lochia ceased (usually 4–6 weeks); return of menstruation if non-lactating (within ∼6–8 weeks); breast-feeding/breast engorgement; bladder function; plans for contraception; rubella status and need for vaccination; ? coping with baby; mood.

Examination: weight (should have lost much of weight gained); BP; MSU (glucose/UTI); abdominal palpation (involution); episiotomy/surgical wounds; ? breast examination (abscesses, etc.).

Investigations: swab lochia if persistant or foul smelling/bloodstained, ? cervical smear if necessary, ? FBC if suspicion anaemia.

Baby's first health review: growth, physical development, vision, hearing, movement, hips.

Reference ranges

Plasma estradiol 17-β
Follicular 110–370 pmol/l
Periovulatory 370–1470 pmol/l
Luteal 180–550 pmol/l
Postmenopausal 20–70 pmol/l

Plasma progesterone
Follicular 0.6–2.9 nmol/l
Luteal 9.5–95 nmol/l
Postmenopausal 0.1–1 nmol/l

Urine assay pregnanediol
Follicular 0–1.6 μmol/24 hour
Luteal > 6 μmol/24 hour
Postmenopausal 0.4–2.8 μmol/24 hour

Urine total oestrogen—non-pregnant
Follicular 25–105 nmol/24 hour
Mid-cycle 140–350 nmol/24 hour
Luteal 105–350 nmol/24 hour

Plasma testosterone
0.7–2.8 nmol/l

Serum FSH
Follicular 3–16 u/l
Mid-cycle 12–27 u/l
Luteal 2–16 u/l
Postmenopausal 40–250 u/l

Serum LH
Follicular 3–45 u/l
Mid-cycle 45–300 u/l
Luteal 3–45 u/l
Postmenopausal 49–128 u/l

Prolactin
25–396 u/l

Breast Feeding

1. **How is lactation initiated in puerperium?**
   - Following delivery, fall in oestrogen & progesterone
   - High prolactin levels signal alveolar cells to start producing/secreting milk.
   - Suckling leads to reflex surge in prolactin secretion, c̄ milk let down, & oxytocin release
   - Oxytocin causes contract. of myoepithelial cells c̄ passage of milk into lactiferous ducts & sinuses.

2. **What is composition of human breast milk?**
   - water
   - protein (casein, lactalbumin, lactoferrin, immunoglobulins)
   - fat
   - carbohydrates
   - minerals
   - trace elements
   - vitamins
   - enzymes
   - hormones

3. **Advantages?**
   - cost
   - convenience
   - freshness
   - sterility
   - correct temp.
   - lactional amenorrhoea
   - ideal composition
   - anti-infective prop.
   - portability
   - mat-infant bond.
   - uterine involution

4) How is full lactation in preg. prevented?

- Progesterone interferes c̄ binding of prolactin to its receptors ā glandular tissue of breast

5) What is the name of fluid produced in breast in 1st few days after delivery?

- Colostrum

Consists of?

- desquamated epithelial cells &
- transudate from maternal serum - which has a high content of antibodies